CHINESE
MEDICINE BIBLE

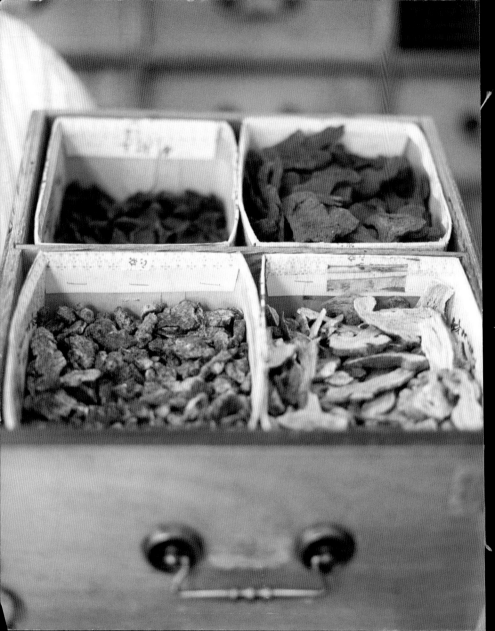

CHINESE MEDICINE BIBLE

The definitive guide to holistic healing

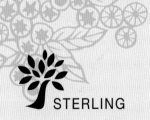

STERLING

New York / London
www.sterlingpublishing.com

STERLING and the distinctive Sterling logo are
registered trademarks of Sterling Publishing Co., Inc.

10 9 8 7 6 5 4 3 2 1

Published by Sterling Publishing Co., Inc.
387 Park Avenue South, New York, NY 10016

First published in Great Britain in 2010 by
Godsfield, a division of Octopus Publishing Group Ltd.

Distributed in Canada by Sterling Publishing
c/o Canadian Manda Group, 165 Dufferin Street,
Toronto, Ontario, Canada M6K 3H6

Printed and bound in China

Sterling ISBN: 978-1-4027-8091-2

For information about custom editions, special sales,
premium and corporate purchases, please contact
Sterling Special Sales Department at 800-805-5489
or specialsales@sterlingpublishing.com.

Chinese pictograms are generally transliterated
into English using the pinyin or Wade-Giles
systems. These are slightly different: *qi* in pinyin,
for example, is *ch'i* in Wade-Giles. The Chinese
use different positions of the tongue in Mandarin
to alter the sounds of words giving entirely
different meanings for each apparently similar
transliteration: diacritical marks are generally
used in pinyin to guide pronunciation and thus
meaning. For simplicity in this book where
Chinese names are given in the text they are
usually written in the pinyin form but without
accents and these are only included where there
could be confusion. For clarity where a word used
in English implies a Chinese interpretation (as in
the names of the body organs or syndromes), it is
given a capital letter

This book is not intended as an alternative to
personal medical advice. The reader should consult
a physician in all matters relating to health and
particularly in respect of any symptoms that may
require diagnosis or medical attention. While the
advice and information are believed to be accurate
and true at the time of going to press, neither the
author nor the publisher can accept any legal
responsibility or liability for any error or omissions
that may have been made.

CONTENTS

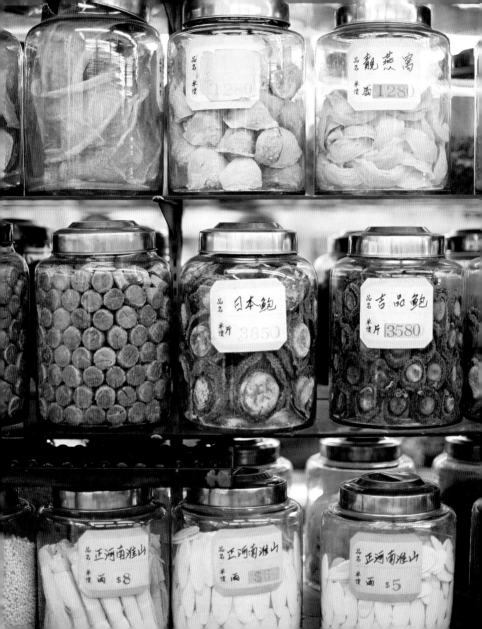

FOREWORD

Traditional Chinese medical theory has been based on the characters of nature's five elements. The five elements, *yin* and *yang* and various Channels have been used to explain the phenomena of the human being and provide the basis for treatment.

The principles of traditional Chinese medical diagnosis and treatment include observing diseases by taking the human body as a whole and treating each individual as unique, comprehensively analysing data gained from all diagnostic methods and combining the diagnosis of diseases with differentiation of syndromes. Chinese medicine can detect subtle imbalances in the body, therefore providing treatment before the disease develops, so it is an excellent form of preventive medicine.

Traditional Chinese medicine has developed over thousands of years in China, but Western society only became familiar with Chinese Medicine in the late 20th century and most books were written in Chinese. This book by Penelope Ody presents a full picture of Chinese medicine and its engagement with health and diseases. I believe that the book offers a well-rounded window into the way Chinese medicine understands the world and body, and provides enormous material not only for those who practice Chinese medicine, but also for those who are interested in an alternative way of keeping well.

May all those who come into Chinese medicine have their lives protected and their diseases healed.

Kezheng Liang, Dr. of TCM

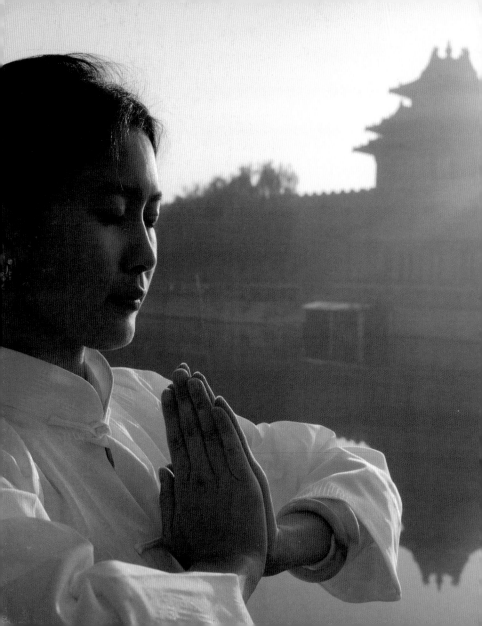

Part 1

THE THEORY
OF CHINESE
MEDICINE

FROM MYTH TO MODERN MEDICINE

Chinese medicine begins with myth—around 5,000 years ago there lived two great emperors, the Yellow, Huang Di, and the Red, Yan Di. The Yellow Emperor taught mankind to weave silk, play musical scales and practice the martial arts while the Red Emperor was the first to cultivate the five grains (millet, rye, sesame, and two types of wheat), introducing agriculture to the world and earning the title Divine Farmer or Shen Nong.

Shen Nong was the first to make tea, and he also tasted hundreds of plants and minerals to discover their medicinal properties, so tradition says, because he had a transparent body and could see the effects on himself of the various herbal brews. He is claimed as the author of China's first herbal, the *Shen Nong Ben Cao Jing* (*The Divine Farmer's Herb Classic*), although the book itself was compiled in more recent historic times.

Huang Di, meanwhile, was also helping mankind learn more about medicine; with the help of his physician Qi Bo, he is credited with the *Huang Di Nei Jing Su Wen* (usually abbreviated to *Nei Jing*)—the *Yellow Emperor's Classic of Internal Medicine*, believed to have been written around 1000 BCE. The *Nei Jing* discusses the nature of *yin* and *yang* as well as the theory of the five elements and their impact on the universe, human health, and bodily functions. The book was annotated and expanded many times

Shen Nong, the Divine Farmer, identified hundreds of herbs.

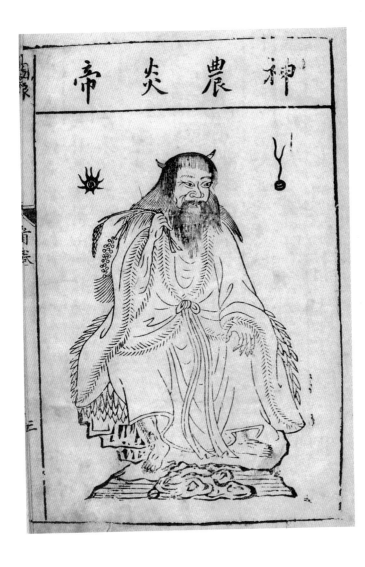

over the centuries with surviving texts dating from the 14th century CE.

The theories explained in the *Nei Jing* form the basis of traditional Chinese medicine as it is still practiced today, while the 365 herbs, minerals, and animal parts listed in Shen Nong's herbal are among the most important Chinese remedies in current use.

CENTURIES OF PRACTICE

While Chinese medicine began with myth, its practice has been recorded for centuries: around 400 BCE Qin Yueren first described Chinese diagnostic techniques; acupuncture needles have been found in Han Dynasty tombs (206 BCE–CE 220); Tao Honjing in the 6th century CE expanded Shen Nong's list of herbs to 730 remedies; while the great herbalist Li Shi Zhen (1518–1573) published his *Ben Cao Gang Mu* in the 1590s, listing some 1,892 remedies. Over the centuries the traditional theories were gradually expanded, with medical scholars producing detailed texts on everything from treating feverish diseases and epidemics to childhood disorders, skin problems, or acupuncture.

While the formalized theories and remedies credited to Huang Di and Shen Nong were familiar to the affluent ruling classes of Chinese society, most people depended on folk medicine and itinerant physicians so that healthcare in remote regions remained extremely basic.

All this began to change in the 18th century with the arrival of European missionaries and traders. Western-style dissections of corpses—previously banned—demonstrated the true function of the various organs. Chinese doctors began to travel abroad to study this new medicine with the first student, Huang Kuan, arriving at Edinburgh's noted medical school in the 1850s. By the beginning of the 20th century China had its own colleges teaching Western medicine and traditional techniques were largely dismissed as unscientific.

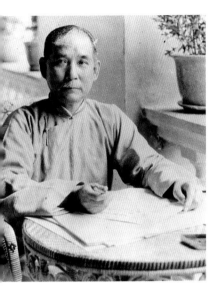

Sun Yat-sen was a western-trained doctor who frowned on traditional medicine.

imposed restrictions on the traditional techniques by banning new colleges and strictly controlling practice. The strategy met with considerable resistance and compromise became inevitable; research into Chinese remedies was undertaken to demonstrate their efficacy in scientific terms, and attempts were made to merge Western and traditional Chinese medical theories.

Under Mao Zedong in the 1950s, new traditional Chinese medicine colleges were established in Shanghai, Liaoning, Zhejiang, and Henan, along with many factories producing pills and powders based on traditional prescriptions.

Today, traditional Chinese medicine is available throughout China, as is our familiar Western medicine, with patients able to choose treatments from either discipline—or indeed, to opt for the many regional folk cures which still survive.

TRADITIONAL MEDICINE IN A MODERN AGE

Perhaps the most famous of China's Western-style doctors was Sun Yat-sen (1866–1925), who led the revolution that overthrew the last Qing emperor in 1911. Sun had studied medicine in Guangzhou (Canton) and Hong Kong and practiced at a Macao hospital before taking to politics. He was a keen advocate of Western medicine, and the new Nationalist government

THE NATURAL WORLD AND THE FIVE-ELEMENT THEORY

Traditional Chinese medicine developed from a very different view of the world to that which we hold today. Some ancient Greek philosophers argued that everything was composed of four core elements—earth, air, fire, and water—but the Chinese imagined a world derived from five processes: wood (*mù*), fire (*huǒ*), earth (*tǔ*), metal (*jīn*), and water (*shuǐ*) known collectively as *wǔxíng* or *wǔ xíng* (usually translated as movements or elements).

Unlike the Western elements these movements are not fixed substances but are more active. Wood, for example, is associated with growing, while fire is transforming or consuming.

The five elements are closely related and reflect the seasonal changes those early thinkers saw in the world around them. Winter rains (water), gave rise to new growth in spring (wood), which in turn would be burnt in the scorching heat of a central Asian summer (fire), to create ashes (earth), from which metal ores could be extracted, metal in its turn is cold causing the water vapor in warm air to appear as condensation.

Each element therefore gives rise to the next in the cycle—traditionally described as a mother-son relationship—so water is seen as the mother of wood while metal gives birth to wood. The strength or weakness of each element also affects that of its neighbors: too little water and the green shoots in spring will not appear, too little fire and there will be no ashes to strengthen earth, and so on. In the

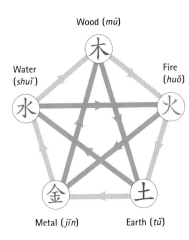

Wood (*mù*)

Water (*shuǐ*)

Fire (*huǒ*)

Metal (*jīn*)

Earth (*tǔ*)

The five-element system

of roots can divide and move earth, while earth, in its turn, will muddy water. There are reverse restraints, too, since wood will absorb water which also rusts metal, while metal breaks up earth which can smother fire and fire can, of course burn wood.

Having created a world view in which everything is linked to five core elements the Chinese then extended the model to take in every aspect of life: five seasons, five directions, five colors, five tastes, five sounds, and so on.

They also identified five *zang* or solid organs in the body and five *fu* or hollow organs. These organs are conceptual and bear little relation to accepted anatomy and physiology. The relationship between these organs is also the same as that between the elements so the Liver is seen as the mother of the Heart, while the Kidneys are the mother of the Liver. Equally the Heart (fire) will control the Lungs (metal) while Kidneys (water) can control the

reverse direction there are also controlling influences: wood will absorb water, and water can rust metal, metal can break up earth which will smother fire, while fire burns wood.

CONTROLS AND RESTRAINTS

Each element also exerts control over others elsewhere in the cycle: water, obviously, can put out fire while fire will melt metal, metal can chop wood while wood in the form

FIVE ELEMENT CONNECTIONS

	Wood	Fire	Earth
Direction	East	South	Center
Color	Green	Red	Yellow
Season	Spring	Summer	Late Summer
Climate	Wind	Hot	Dampness
Solid or zang organs	Liver	Heart	Spleen
Hollow or fu	Gall Bladder	Small Intestine	Stomach
Sense organs/openings	Eyes/Sight	Tongue/Speech	Mouth/Taste
Emotion	Anger	Joy/Fright	Worry
Taste	Sour	Bitter	Sweet or Acrid
Tissues	Tendon/Nails	Blood vessels/Complexion	Muscles/Lips
Sound	Shouting	Laughing	Singing
Smell	Rancid	Burnt	Fragrant
Secretions	Tears	Sweat	Saliva
Spiritual aspects	Soul (hun)	Spirit (shén)	Intention (yì)
Fingers	Index	Middle	Thumb
Lifecycle	Birth	Youth	Adulthood

Metal	Water
West	North
White	Black
Autumn	Winter
Dryness	Cold
Lung	Kidney
Large Intestine	Bladder Urinary
Nose/Smell	Ears/Hearing
Sadness/Grief	Fear
Pungent	Salty
Skin/Body hair	Bone/Head hair
Weeping	Groaning
Rotten	Putrid
Mucus	Urine
Vitality (po)	Determination (zhi)
Ring	Little
Old age	Death

Heart (fire). Illness in one organ can thus be traced to a weakness or over-controlling action by a related organ. If water is weak, for example, it will fail to control fire, which becomes over-exuberant and attacks metal; or in organ terms, weak Kidneys fail to control the Heart, which then damages the Lungs, so a respiratory disorder such as asthma may in some cases be treated with kidney tonics.

Other aspects of the five-element relationships also affect health and diagnosis: a craving for or dislike of sour tastes may suggest Liver imbalance or excessive grief may lead to Lung weakness.

OPPOSITES IN EQUILIBRIUM —YIN AND YANG

The concept of *yin* and *yang* is central to Chinese medical theory and describes how opposing forces can be inter-connected and inter-dependent while present in all things. One common analogy is a mountain—one side bathed in bright sunlight and the other in deep shadow creating two very different environments within one totality. This single entity containing two opposing forces is characterized by the traditional Taoist *taijitu* diagram—*taijitu* means "diagram of ultimate power."

Yang is often described in the West as representing masculine energies while *yin* is seen as softer and more feminine, but this is a vast over-simplification. *Yin-yang* is not so much an actual entity or force but, like the five elements in the five-element model, it represents processes rather than actual things. It is a more dynamic interaction that is always present and changing rather than an absolute: above/below; outside/inside; strong/weak; dry/damp; hot/cold and so on. *Yang* can be represented by fire: upward moving, bright, warm, active, exciting; while *yin* is water: sinking downward, dim, cold, passive, inhibiting. Both are, however, always present: hot summer may be more *yang* in character but *yin* is still present in cooler nights while winter is *yin* but still contains some sunny *yang* days.

While *yin* and *yang* are opposites and sometimes said to be in dynamic equilibrium, they are also held in balance: one cannot exist without the other and if the balance is tilted

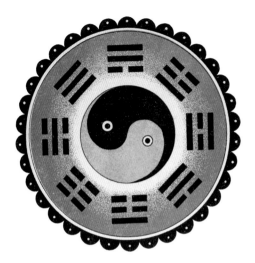

then there can be problems. Within Chinese medicine body parts and functions are seen as more or less *yin* or *yang* although all contain aspects of both.

The Taoist *bagua* symbol shows the *taijitu* surrounded by the eight trigrams representing the fundamental principles of reality.

Substances—passive, unchanging—are seen as more *yin*, while functions—active, changing—are more *yang*. The solid *zang* organs that are associated with storage are thus more *yin* in character, while the hollow *fu* organs that have functions associated with transforming are therefore *yang*. The outside of the body is more *yang* while the inside is more *yin*; the upper half more *yang*, the lower parts more *yin*. Thus the Lungs—*zang* and *yin*—will be slightly more *yang* in character than the Kidneys (also *zang* and *yin*) because they are in the upper part of the body (*yang*) while the Kidneys are lower down (*yin*).

CHARACTERISTICS OF *YIN* AND *YANG*

Yin	Yang
Water	Fire
Dark	Light
Cold	Hot
Passive	Active
Inside	Outside
Slow	Rapid
Right	Left
Dim	Bright
Downward	Upward
Substance	Function
Matter	Energy

MAINTAINING BALANCE

Within the body, the relationship between *yin* and *yang* is constantly changing; sitting indoors, quietly reading a book sees us in a more *yin* mode, while energetically digging the garden on a sunny afternoon is definitely a *yang*-promoting activity.

In health these changes are normal and easily managed; however, in illness or disease the mutual restraint of the opposing forces can become out of control leading to serious

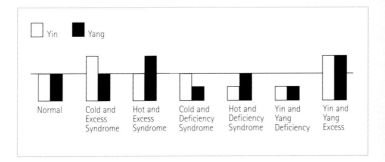

imbalance. Identifying these imbalances is an important aspect of Chinese diagnostics with four possible scenarios for the imbalance. Two involve over-activity leading to Excess disorders and two under-activity, leading to Deficiency syndromes.

EXCESS AND DEFICIENCY

If *yin* is in excess then it can damage *yang* and cause Cold and Excess disorders, while if *yang* is over-active it can lead to Hot and Excess syndromes. If *yin* is weak then *yang* is in apparent excess but this is actually a *yin* Deficiency problem rather than one of surplus *yang* and the result is a Hot and Deficiency syndrome, while if the reverse is true then there is a Cold and Deficiency problem.

In addition, there may be cases where both *yin* and *yang* are Deficient or where they are both in Excess, giving rise to two further possibilities for imbalance.

Obviously in diagnosis it is essential to reach the right conclusion; apparent Cold symptoms could be due to weak *yang* —Cold and Deficiency—or over-active *yin* (Cold and Excess). In the first case treatment would be focused on strengthening *yang*, and in the second on controlling over-exuberant *yin*. However, if the wrong treatment was given, for example, reducing *yin* in a Deficiency disorder, then the syndrome could progress to general *yin-yang* weakness and even greater debility.

ZANG ORGANS

To the ancient Chinese the body contained five *zang* or solid organs—Heart, Liver, Spleen, Lung, and Kidneys. These were said to resemble the solidness of the Earth and were associated with storage so are more *yin* in character. It is important to remember that these organs are not the same as our modern anatomical and physiological concepts: they embrace related systems and include spiritual and emotional aspects as well as physical entities.

The *zang* organs each have an associated hollow organ—the *fu* organs—which are involved with transformation and activity, so are more *yang* in character. The *zang* and *fu* organs are linked by meridians or acupuncture channels (see pages 32–35). Each organ also has an associated fundamental substance such as Blood or *qi* (which is translated as life-force or breath). All these connections relate to the five-element model).

THE HEART

The Heart (*xin*) is generally regarded as the most important or "emperor" of the *zang* organs and is associated with thought and intellect. This is consistent with other ancient medical traditions such as Ayurveda in India where the heart is closely linked to spiritual and emotional activity.

The Heart is believed to control all life processes and coordinates the activities of all the other *zang-fu* organs. In addition it:

- governs the Blood circulation and vessels
- controls mental activities
- stores the Spirit
- is seen in the condition of the complexion
- is linked to the tongue

Rather than regarding the heart as a mechanical pump, the Chinese maintain that blood flows through the arteries and veins because of the power of Heart *qi*. When this is strong and abundant it can be felt as a smooth and forceful pulse; if Heart *qi* is weak then so too is the pulse.

Mental activity also comes under the Heart's dominion: in Chinese terminology this activity includes a wide range of life processes not just perception and thought. In contrast, the brain is simply regarded as a place to receive and store impressions. In Chinese the word for Heart and mind—*xin*—is the same. The Heart is also said to store the Spirit (*shén*) which is sometimes equated with awareness. Several herbal remedies are also described as calming the Spirit and are used to ease mental and emotional upsets which can be linked to Heart disorders.

Because of the strong link between the blood vessels and the Heart, the condition of the Heart is said to be seen in the complexion: a glowing, healthy complexion signifies a healthy Heart while a pale, dull face suggests some weakness. Chinese theory also maintains that we can taste foods because the tongue is supplied with Heart *qi* and is the body opening of the Heart.

THE LIVER

The Liver (*gan*) is sometimes referred to as the "general" of the *zang* organs and works with the Heart to control the Blood supply. The ancient Chinese believed that Blood traveled through the vessels when the body was active but during rest it was stored in the Liver, so it was called the "Reservoir of Blood." This association of the Liver with Blood is why in Chinese theory the Liver is also closely linked to the menstrual cycle. Key functions of the Liver are to:

- store Blood
- regulate the flow of *qi*
- store the Soul
- control the tendons

Healthy pink nails are said to indicate strong Liver energy.

- it can also be seen in the nails and is linked to the eyes

In traditional Chinese medicine the Liver is said to favour a smooth flow of *qi* and has an aversion to stagnancy. A smooth *qi* flow helps to regulate emotional activities, while stagnation or obstruction leads to moodiness, anger, and depression. It also ensures normal digestive function: for the Spleen and Stomach to function properly a smooth flow of *qi* is essential, with irregularity causing dysfunction such as indigestion or jaundice. A smooth *qi* flow from the Liver is also important for the Triple Burner (*san jiao* see page 31)—a mysterious concept to Westerners but important for controlling body fluids.

In traditional Chinese theory it is believed that the Spirit resides in the Heart during the day and the Liver at night when we sleep, when its state can be assessed by dreams, which is why the Liver is said to "store the

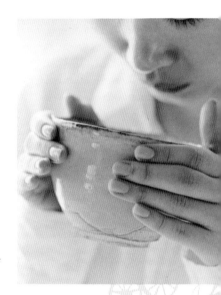

Soul." Spirit itself divides further into *po*—the animal or physical soul that lives in the Lung and controls physical energies; and *hun*—a more ethereal or spiritual aspect of soul that is stored in the Liver and controls both conscious and unconscious thought.

The Liver also controls the tendons so aching knees, where there are a great many tendons, can suggest a Liver imbalance. The nails are believed to indicate the state of Liver energies and health with strong, pink nails implying a strong Liver. In conventional medicine pale fingernails often indicate iron-deficient anemia, whereas the Chinese see this as evidence of a weakened Liver and thus failure to store Blood efficiently. The Liver's role in storing Blood is also said to be one reason why it is linked to the eyes with Deficient Liver Blood leading to poor vision or night blindness; dry eyes and conjunctivitis are similarly linked to weaknesses in the Liver or Liver meridian.

THE SPLEEN

In Western medicine the Spleen (*pi*) filters old red blood cells from our blood and stores blood, and is part of the immune system. In Chinese theory, the Spleen (*pi*) is mainly concerned with digestive function and is responsible for the assimilation and distribution of nutrients and water. The Spleen is said to:
- control digestion
- control the limbs and flesh
- keep Blood in the blood vessels
- store intention or determination
- be linked to the mouth and reflected in the lips

If the Spleen is working well, then "food essence" will be efficiently distributed to the Lungs and Heart, from where it is sent to the rest of the body so that muscles and tissues will be well-formed. The Spleen plays a similar role in managing water distribution through the body, extracting it from food and drink and sending it to the Lungs, Heart, and Urinary Bladder. When Spleen *qi* is strong, Blood is kept within the blood vessels, if *qi* is weak then the Blood can escape to form hemorrhages or subcutaneous bleeding.

Just as the Heart and Liver have a spiritual dimension so too does the Spleen, storing *yi*, which is intention or will power and helps us to make necessary changes in our lives. Spleen weakness or damage can lead to mental confusion, indecisiveness or poor memory.

The mouth is linked to the Spleen—not only is it connected through the muscles, but it is also the source of the food which the Spleen processes. Its body opening is the lips: red, lustrous lips suggest that nutrients are being processed and distributed well, while pale lips and poor appetite suggest Spleen malfunction.

THE LUNG

The Lung (*fei*) is the "prime minister," managing air and water within the body and, importantly, controlling *qi* flow. Traditionally the Lung is aid to:

- control *qi* and respiration
- maintain the downward flow of body fluids
- regulate water circulation
- store vitality or animal soul
- be linked to the nose and is seen in the skin and body hair

In Chinese theory, as indeed with yoga practices from India, breath is linked to vital energy so it is understandable that the ancients linked the Lung to the flow of *qi*. The Lung is especially associated with *wèi qi*, a form of defence energy that can be equated with the immune system. Lung *qi* is believed to disperse *wèi qi* and Body Fluids to help warm and nourish the skin and muscles. The skin is especially associated with the Lung, with the sweat pores known in Chinese medicine as the "portal of energy:" production of sweat is under the control of the *wèi qi*.

Lung *qi* has a downward direction so it ensures that water and body fluids travel throughout the body and down to the urinary bladder for excretion. Any weakness in Lung *qi* can thus lead to edema or fluid retention.

The Lung also stores an aspect of soul—*po*, the animal soul that manifests as vitality. Sorrow and anxiety can damage this vitality and cause stagnation of Lung *qi* leading to depression and dejection. As one would expect, the nose is the body opening of the Lung with the sense of smell also dependent on Lung *qi*.

THE KIDNEY

As one might expect the Chinese believe that Kidney (*shén*) is responsible for regulating water in the body. An equally important role, however, is to store the vital essence or *jīng*—one of the five fundamental substances and the source of living organisms. The Kidney also promotes growth and development of the body and plays an important role in reproduction. Its main functions are to:

● store vital essence
● produce bone marrow
● regulate water in the body
● help to co-ordinate respiration
● store determination

The condition of the Kidney can be seen in the head hair and it is linked to the ears and genitals.

In Chinese theory the Kidney has an important role to play in water metabolism by helping the Lung to co-ordinate respiration by directing the *qi* downward. Strong Kidney *qi* leads to even, regular breathing while weak Kidney *qi* impairs inhalation

leading to "Deficiency-type" asthma. Water metabolism is also associated with Body Fluids and the Kidney is responsible for sending clear Fluids upward to circulate in the tissues while turbid Fluids are transformed into sweat and urine for excretion.

The vital essence (see pages 42–45) stored in the Kidney has many functions including the creation of bone marrow, both that found in the large bones of the body and a "spinal marrow" believed to fill the spinal chord and brain.

Determination or will (*zhi*) is also stored in the Kidney: strong Kidney *qi* therefore leads to good memory, vigor, wisdom, and well-developed skills. If Kidney *qi* is weak then the memory is poor, spirits are low and there is a lack of aspiration. Meridians link the Kidney to the ears, genitals and anus so it is also responsible for hearing, reproduction, and excretion. Kidney energy declines with age so signs of ageing—such as balding head hair, and hearing loss—are also linked to Kidney weakness.

FU ORGANS

The *fu* or hollow organs are associated with transformation rather than storage so are thus more *yang* in character than the *zang* organs. One of the *fu* organs is linked to each of the *zang* organ with a sixth—the Triple Burner—a more nebulous entity.

THE SMALL INTESTINE

The Small Intestine (*xiao chang*) forms a *zang-fu* pair with the Heart and is said to have the function of "receiving and containing" water and food which has been digested in the Stomach. It "differentiates the usable from the unusable" sorting the usable materials—described as "clear"— that are eventually transported as nutrients or "food essence" to other parts of the body while the unusable or turbid are sent onward as solid wastes to the Large Intestine or or as liquid to the Kidney and Urinary Bladder for excretion. Although the terminology may be different the Small Intestine's function is thus much as one would expect from conventional Western physiology.

THE GALL BLADDER

In Western medicine a key function of the gallbladder is to store around 50 ml (2 fl oz) of bile produced by the liver: this is then released to help digest fats. In Chinese theory bile is seen instead as surplus Liver *qi* so plays a part in promoting the smooth flow of *qi* and Blood. The Gall Bladder (*dan*) is also associated with decisiveness, activity and decision-making; in contrast weak Gall Bladder energy leads to dithering and lack of determination.

THE STOMACH

Paired with the Spleen, the Stomach (*wéi*) is primarily involved in taking in and transforming food into chyme, the semi-fluid mass of part-digested food that the stomach sends onward to the intestines. In Chinese theory, the efficiency of this onward movement is related to the strength of the Stomach *qi* so the vigor of all the *zang-fu* organs depends on the abundance of Stomach *qi*. The Stomach's activity complements that of the Spleen:

the Spleen maintains the upward flow of *qi*, while the Stomach sends digested food downward. The Spleen is involved in the upward transportation of water so is said to be clear with an aversion to Dampness, while the Stomach is turbid so prefers Dampness.

The Stomach, as in Western anatomy, plays a major role in digesting food.

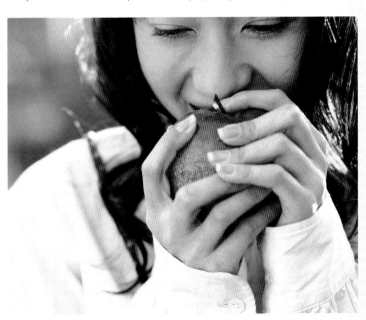

THE LARGE INTESTINE

The Large Intestine (*da chang*) is linked to the Lung and is where the unusable or turbid material from the Small Intestine is transformed into solid waste for excretion and water which is reabsorbed. These functions mirror the Western understanding.

THE URINARY BLADDER

The Urinary Bladder (*pang guang*) is linked to the Kidney and stores and excretes urine. In Chinese theory, the Kidney separates clear and turbid Fluids and the Urinary Bladder removes the unusable turbid Fluids from the body. Urinary function is

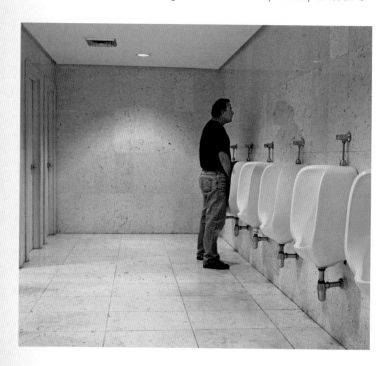

said to be controlled by Kidney *yang* so if this is weak there may be increased frequency of urination or a need to urinate at night. The Chinese say that when Kidney energy is strong, there is no need for frequent urination.

THE TRIPLE BURNER

The sixth *fu* organ is the Triple Burner (*san jiao*) which is a concept dating back to the *Yellow Emperor's Classic of Internal Medicine* (at least 1000 BCE). It attempts to describe the digestive function and the separation of clear from turbid Fluid. It is the basis and controller for the circulation of Body Fluids and occupies the entire torso—from the base of the tongue to the anus.

The Upper Burner or *shang jiao* (from tongue to diaphragm) is linked to the function of Heart and

In Chinese theory poor Kidney energy is associated with the need for frequent urination.

Lung, and include transmitting *qi* and nutrients, warming the body, nourishing the skin and spreading the defence energy or *wèi qi*.

The Middle Burner or *zhong jiao* (from diaphragm to navel) reflects the functions of the Spleen and Stomach and is mainly concerned with digesting foods, absorbing and transporting nutrients, and producing various Body Fluids.

The Lower Burner or *xia jiao* (from navel to anus) reflects the function of the Kidney, Large Intestine, Small Intestine, and Urinary Bladder in separating clear and turbid Fluids and managing excretion. The Liver is also associated with the lower *jiao*, with the smooth flow of Liver *qi* ensuring orderly functioning of the *san jiao*.

The *san jiao* is sometimes paired with the Pericardium which can be defined as a sixth *zang* organ although the classic Chinese texts tend to see this Pericardium-Triple Burner pairing as a subset of the Small Intestine.

MERIDIANS— THE CHANNEL SYSTEM

Alongside the *zang-fu* organs, traditional Chinese anatomy also comprises the Channel system—a network of pathways through the body that link the organs and distribute *qi* and other fundamental substances. Keeping these intangible routes, sometimes called meridians, clear of obstructions is vital to good health.

In the West these Channels have become known through acupuncture treatments, with needles used at specific points to stimulate or ease the flow of *qi*. In Chinese theory, however, they have a wider role: herbs are often defined in terms of the meridians they affect while numerous disease syndromes are connected to various Channel afflictions. The concept involves picturing the body as three concentric cylinders. The outer cylinder is home to the flesh and joints, the middle cylinder is where the principal or primary channels run and the innermost cylinder houses the *zang-fu* organs.

The 12 primary Channels (*jing mai*) are linked to the *zang-fu* organs including the Pericardium and Triple Burner; six of these Channels are *yang* and six are *yin*. They form six pairs with those associated on the front of the limbs known as *taiyin* and *yangming*, those on the back of the limbs as *shaoyin* and *taiyang*, and those mid-way known as *jueyin* and *shaoyang*. Many health problems are specifically associated with disharmonies or blockages within these important Channels.

Acupuncture has been used in China since the days of the Yellow Emperor.

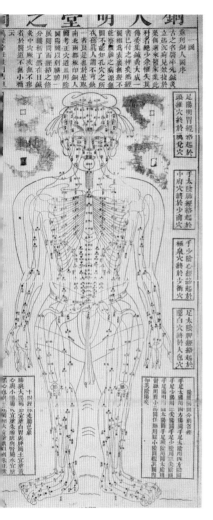

SECONDARY CHANNELS

There are eight secondary Channels (*qi jing ba mai*) that help communications between pairs of primary Channels to ensure a steady flow of *qi* and Blood. The two most important of these are the Governing Vessel (*du mai*) and the Conception Vessel (*ren mai*). The *du mai* runs from the anus, up the spine, across the crown of the head, and ends inside the upper lip; it governs the *yang* Channels. The *ren mai* governs the *yin* Channels and in women is closely associated with pregnancy; it runs up the front of the body starting at the uterus or pelvic cavity to the inside of the lower lip.

The other six Channels are the:

- Penetrating Vessel *(chong mai)*, that communicates with the main Channels
- Girdle Vessel *(dai mai)* which runs around the waist like a belt and binds all the Channels together
- *Yin* Heel (*yin qiao jing*) associated with excess sleep
- *Yang* Heel (*yang qiao jing*) associated with insomnia

THE 12 MAIN CHANNELS AND ASSOCIATED HEALTH PROBLEMS

Affected organ	Meridian	Typical signs of disharmony
Heart	Hand *shaoyin*	Heart pain, palpitations, insomnia, night sweats
Small Intestine	Hand *taiyang*	Deafness, lower abdominal pain, and distention
Liver	Foot *jueyin*	Low back or abdominal pain, mental disturbances, hiccoughs
Bladder	Foot *shaoyang*	Headache, blurred vision, shoulder pain
Spleen	Foot *taiyin*	Flatulence, vomiting, upper abdominal pain
Stomach	Foot *yangming*	Abdominal bloating, vomiting, abdominal pain
Lung	Hand *taiyin*	Coughs, asthma, chest pains
Large Intestine	Hand *yangming*	Toothache, sore throats, neck pains
Kidney	Foot *shaoyin*	Impotence, weakness in the lower limbs, increased frequency of urination
Urinary Bladder	Foot *taiyang*	Urinary retention, nasal catarrh, headache, back pain
Pericardium	Hand *jueyin*	Heart pain, poor concentration, palpitations
San jiao	Hand *shaoyang*	Abdominal bloating, deafness, tinnitus, urinary dysfunction

- *Yin* Tie (*yin wie jing*) ties together the *yin* channels, connecting and regulating them
- *Yang* Tie (*yang wei jing*) ties the *yang* Channels together in the same way

OTHER CHANNELS

In addition, there are 12 distinct Channels (*bei jing*), that improve communications between *yin* and *yang* Channels and co-ordinate the exterior and the interior of the body, and 15 connecting Channels that are also involved in communication: 13 of these are linked to the primary Channels (the Spleen meridian has two) and two are associated with the *ren mai* and *du mai*.

There are also 12 tendon-muscle channels located in the superficial tissues and influence how *qi* flows in the muscles rather than the internal organs. Finally there are countless small collateral Channels throughout the body that run on the surface and help *qi* and Blood to circulate

between the interior and exterior Channels.

On each Channel are a number of points where *qi* is carried to the surface and where acupuncture or other treatments can help to regulate the flow of both *qi* and Blood. There are some 361 points on the 14 main channels, with perhaps 2,000 or more points in total on all Channels and collaterals although only around 150 are regularly used in acupuncture treatments. (Detailed diagrams showing the key Channels can be found on pages 224–241.)

FUNDAMENTAL SUBSTANCES

Along with the five *zang* and five *fu* organs, the Chinese five-element model also identifies five fundamental substances: *qi*, *jīng*, *xue*, *jin-ye* and *shèn*—vital life materials on which our health and vitality depends.

VITAL ENERGY

Of the five substances *qi* is perhaps the most familiar: a concept of essential energy that sits comfortably with the traditional Western notion of a vital life force. *Qi* is, however, far more complex, with some 32 different types of *qi* identified in numerous texts. As a whole, the body's *qi* is generally described as upright (*zheng*) or true (*zhen*), which is a sort of undifferentiated *qi* not associated with specific organs or functions. This *qi* has three possible origins:

- Primordial or prenatal (*yuan qi*) is the *qi* we are born with and derives from our parents
- Grain *qi* (*gu qi*) derived from the food we eat
- Nature or air *qi* (*kong qi*) extracted from the air we breathe

Zheng or *zhen qi* (referred to just as *qi*) is made from the mingling of these three different types of *qi* and has five major functions covering: movement; protection; transformation of food; warmth; and retention of the body's substances and organs.

Qi is said to be in constant motion and in normal health these

Kong qi is derived from the air we breath. It is one of the three sources of *qi* in the body.

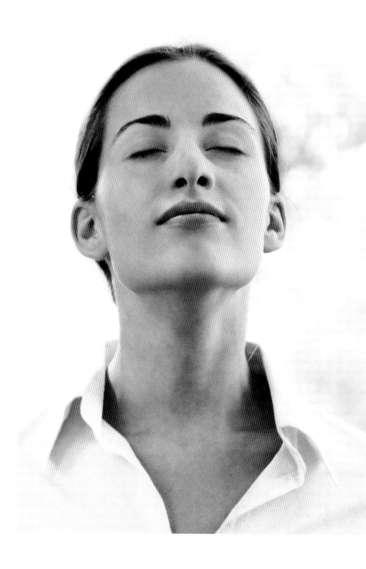

IDENTIFYING DISHARMONIES

Time	Meridians
3–5 am	Lung
5–7 am	Large Intestine
7–9 am	Stomach
9–11 am	Spleen
11 am–1 pm	Heart
1–3 pm	Small Intestine
3–5 pm	Urinary Bladder
5–7 pm	Kidney
7–9 pm	Pericardium
9–11 pm	*San jiao*
11 pm–1 am	Gall Bladder
1–3 am	Liver

movements flow steadily and harmoniously through the meridians. If there is insufficient *qi* or some sort of obstruction then *qi* becomes disordered and ill health follows. In health there is a regular rhythm to this *qi* flow and disharmonies can be identified by the times at which they occur. Waking regularly in the early hours, for example, could suggest some obstruction in energy flow from Liver to Lung.

As well as flowing through the channels, normal *qi* also provides each of the *zang-fu* organs with their own specific *qi* relevant to its particular functions. Other important types nclude *wèi qi* or protective *qi*. This is usually regarded as an aspect of the normal *zheng qi* although it is sometimes described as also derived from grain *qi*. The *wèi qi* can be thought of as an aspect of the immune system defending the body from external attack. The *wèi qi* travels on the surface and exterior parts of the body in skin and muscle where it also regulates body temperature and sweating.

This circulation is largely a daytime phenomenon with the *wèi qi* traveling up the spine, across the head in the morning, down the front of the body during the afternoon to reach the lower spine at night, where it retreats back into the body. Because of this the time of onset of an external disorder is significant in Chinese medicine.

PECTORAL *QI* AND NOURISHING *QI*

While normal *qi* is derived from primordial *qi*, grain *qi* and nature *qi*, the grain *qi* and nature *qi* also combine to produce pectoral *qi* (*zong qi*). This is stored in the chest and its main function is to control the rhythms of respiration and heartbeat making it responsible for the movement of the Blood, the voice, and the strength and regularity of breathing and heartbeat.

Nourishing *qi* (*ying qi*) is largely produced from grain *qi*, which is collected and transformed by the Spleen. This form of energy transforms some of the food we eat into Blood, which carries these nutrients to all parts of the body.

While there are many different types of *qi* there are two main disharmonies that can afflict it leading to ill health: Deficient (*qi xu*), which manifests as various weaknesses; and Stagnant (*qi zhi*) where the flow is impaired interrupting normal function of the affected organs. In Western terms, problems associated with physiological dysfunction of any particular organ would, in Chinese theory, be associated with *qi* problems.

BLOOD

While *xue* is generally translated as Blood in Chinese theory, it indicates a substance with rather more functions than simply carrying oxygen and nutrients to the tissues. *Xue* is also seen as essential for mental activities and circulates not just in the blood vessels, but also in the meridians.

Blood, like post-natal *jīng*, is produced from food. The Stomach and Spleen are believed to process the food leading to production of a pure substance, which is then carried by the Spleen *qi* to the Lungs. In the process this substance begins its conversion into Blood—a process competed by the addition of air in the Lungs. This Blood or *xue* is then propelled through the body by the Heart *qi*. *Qi*—active and therefore *yang* in character—is thus very important for creating and moving Blood, which is liquid and thus *yin* in nature. If *xue* and *qi* are strong then the person will be clear-thinking and vigorous—if not they may lack energy and have problems concentrating. *Xue* is particularly associated with three of the *zang* organs: the Heart, the Liver, and the Spleen.

BLOOD DISORDERS

Health problems associated with Blood fall into two main categories:

If Blood (*xue*) and *qi* are strong then a person will be clear-thinking and vigorous.

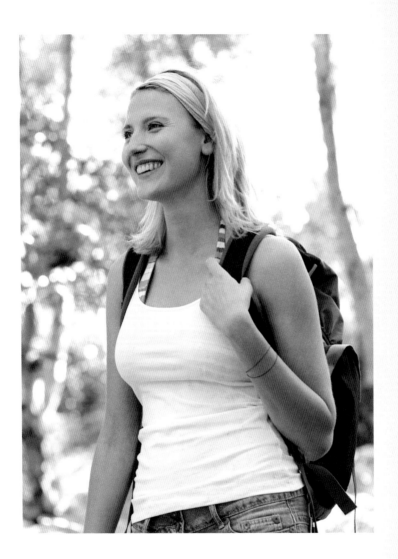

Deficient Blood *(xue xu)*; and Congealed or Stagnant Blood *(xue yu)*. Blood may be Deficient throughout the body—typified by pallor, lethargy, dizziness, and dry skin. In the West this would suggest iron-deficient anemia, although in Chinese theory it would be treated by an herb such as *dang gui* (Chinese angelica), said to nourish the Blood. Alternatively Blood may be Deficient from a specific organ—if the Heart was affected, for example, then there could be irregular heart beat or palpitations.

Stagnant Blood is caused when it is obstructed and no longer flows smoothly through the vessels or the meridians. This may be characterized by sharp stabbing pains and swelling or tumors.

VITAL ESSENCE

Jīng can be translated as "essence" and is the most important of the fundamental substances as it underpins all organic life. Vital essence is stored in the Kidney and derives from two sources: congenital essence *(xian tian zhi jīng)*; and acquired or post-natal essence *(hiu tian zhi jīng)*.

CONGENITAL ESSENCE

The congenital essence, also known as "before heaven," is inherited from one's parents: it is unique, is with us from conception, and is responsible for our growth, make-up and constitution, controlling our reproduction and creativity. Reproductive problems, such as infertility, impotence, or repeated

Congenital essence is with us from birth and is inherited from our parents.

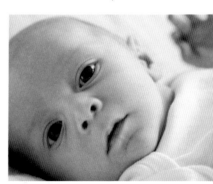

miscarriages, can all be associated in Chinese medicine with weakness of *jīng*. Congenital essence is also fixed; it cannot be expanded or increased and runs down gradually throughout our lifetime. Its loss is associated with the physical signs of ageing— greying hair, deafness, increased urination—which are all linked in the five-element model to the Kidney and water element.

POST-NATAL ESSENCE

This essence is produced by the Spleen from the purified components in our food and water and is known as "after heaven." This essence can help strengthen the vitality of the congenital essence and can itself be improved by good diet and lifestyle. Unlike the fixed "before heaven" component, this part of the total *jīng* can be replenished and can help to compensate for any weaknesses in the inherited congenital *jīng*.

In women the run-down in congenital essence is also marked by the start of the menopause, which in

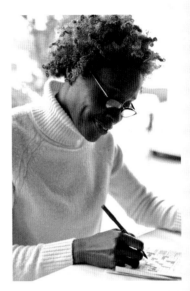

In Chinese theory a woman's reproductive life ends at 49.

Chinese medicine is often treated with Kidney tonics. The original *Yellow Emperor's Classic of Internal Medicine* (the *Nei Jing*) refers to women's lives as occurring in periods of seven years with puberty at age 14, wisdom teeth at 21, and a peak in strength and vitality at 28. By 49 "...the gates of menstruation are no longer open; her body deteriorates, and she is no longer able to bear children."

With men, according to the *Nei Jing*, the life pattern is based on eight-year periods with the final *jīng* run-down starting at 56 when "...his secretion of semen is exhausted, his vitality diminishes, his kidneys deteriorate, and his physical strength reaches its end."

While *qi* is associated with movement, *jīng* is less dynamic, associated more with inner growth and ultimate decline. It is linked to creativity with excessive creative activity rapidly exhausting the limited supply of congenital *jīng*.

As the vital underpinning for organic life, *jīng* can also feed some of the other fundamental substances nurturing *xue* (Blood) and *qi* when need be. *Qi* can then help to energize the Spleen so encouraging production of post-natal essence. *Jīng* is also

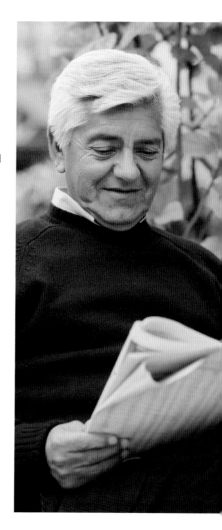

In traditional Chinese theory men reach old age at 56 when "...kidneys deteriorate and physical strength reaches its end."

associated with the production of bone marrow, which ancient Chinese theory also equates with the brain. Brain damage or weaknesses in memory and concentration are also thus associated with *jīng* Deficiency and may be treated with strengthening Kidney tonics. If *qi* is the energetic life force that dictates our vitality and activity, then *jīng* is the physical bedrock that underlies our basic strength and reproduction.

BODY FLUIDS

Jin-ye refers to clear (*jin*) and turbid (*ye*) body fluids and covers all the liquids in the body other than Blood: the category thus includes sweat, urine, saliva, tears, mucus, and gastric juices. These body fluids are derived from food and water and converted by the Stomach and Spleen into *jin* and *ye*. Their function is to moisten, lubricate, and nourish the body with the heavier, turbid fluids supporting the inner parts of the body and the lighter, clear fluids focused on the exterior.

Like Blood, the body fluids are *yin* in nature and any disharmonies manifest as dryness a well as forming part of more general *yin* problems. The clear fluids are also involved in the production of Blood so *jin-ye* weakness can also lead to Deficient Blood problems. The *jin-ye* circulate in the body and come under the control of the Spleen, Lungs, and Kidneys: weaknesses in these organs can also contribute to Deficient Fluid syndromes.

SPIRIT

If *jīng* represents our physical nature and the source of life and *qi* our life force, energy and our ability to move and be active, then *shén* is our spiritual aspect and the vitality of consciousness behind both *jīng* and *qi*. The word is generally translated as "spirit" and is the most nebulous of the five fundamental substances. It is also sometimes translated as "awareness" and is said to be seen in the alert brightness of the eyes when someone is fully conscious of their surroundings, actions and capabilities. If *shén* is weakened then the eyes are said to lackluster and thinking can become muddled.

Like congenital *jīng*, *shén* is something we inherit from our parents, although unlike congenital *jīng* it can be nurtured and encouraged throughout our lives by a healthy lifestyle with time for meditation and exercise therapies.

TANGIBLE ASPECTS

Although referred to as spirit, *shén* is seen in Chinese theory as having more tangible aspects: it exists as a fundamental substance within the body and is part of the body. In the West, body and spirit have been seen as separate entities since the 17th century but in Chinese philosophy this division has never occurred.

Shén disharmonies can manifest as insomnia, confusion or forgetfulness. More severe forms can include speech problems, with incoherent rambling or even, in extreme cases, psychotic illnesses,

violent madness, severe hallucinations, or unconsciousness. Just as *jīng* is stored in the Kidney, so *shén* is stored in the Heart with Heart disharmonies also damaging the spirit. It is not unusual to find people suffering from Heart weakness or irregularity showing signs of *shén* impairment with disordered speech, conversation that jumps from one topic to another with no clear thread or, in severe cases, the sort of manic behavior associated with bouts of dementia.

Shén is not confined to medicine but is an important concept in Chinese philosophy and some sources give it as many as 11 different meanings including god, mind, respect, expression, rule, magic, and caution. It is sometimes translated as soul—but that simply adds further confusion with *hun* (spiritual soul) and *po* (physical soul) (see page 48).

The concept of the *shén* (spirit) goes back to the early Taoists and incorporates such ideas as god and mind.

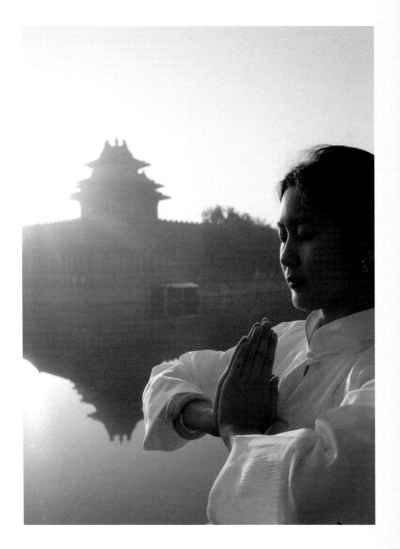

SPIRITUAL ASPECTS

In Chinese medicine many illnesses are seen as having a spiritual dimension and, holistically, this must also be considered in diagnosis and treatment.

The combined spirit of a person—*shén qi*—is said to live in the Heart by day and the Liver by night: during the day its quality can be assessed by the eyes, which in health can be seen as a shining light in the pupils. At night it can be monitored in dreams with a lack of dreams said to indicate a calm and contented Spirit.

Shén qi is variously described in different texts and the terminology can overlap and seem confusing, especially as sources are not always completely consistent in their definitions. In the *Nei Jing*, for example, the terms *qi* and *shén* are sometimes used interchangeably.

FIVE ASPECTS OF SPIRIT

Just as there are five sold organs, five fundamental substances, five hollow organs and so on, there are five defined aspects of spirit: *hun, po, zhi, yi*, and *shén*.

Two contrasting aspects of spirit or soul are *hun* and *po*. *Hun* is a more ethereal or spiritual aspect of soul and controls conscious and unconscious thoughts as well as being associated with moving energies. *Po* is sometimes translated as "animal soul" or "physical soul," and directs physical energies and vitality; it is associated more with substance than energy. *Hun* resides in the Liver and is said to be the part of the soul that survives after death while *po* is stored in the Lung.

Zhi, which resides in the Kidneys, is sometimes translated as animal will or determination but it is associated

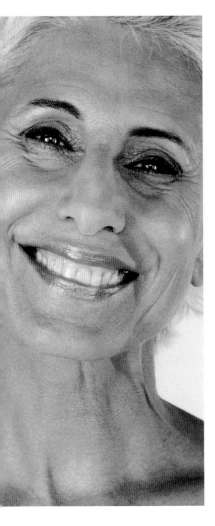

with wants and desires as well as with developing wisdom. *Yi*, stored in the Spleen, controls reflection and intention and is sometimes described as the "consciousness of possibilities." *Yi* makes change possible and in Spleen Deficiency sufferers sometimes lack the ability to make these changes.

The terminology becomes even more confusing with *shén*, which resides in the Heart but is not quite the same as the total *shén qi*, which comprises all five aspects of spirit/soul. In this spiritual context *shén* is associated with propriety and correctness so that disharmonies of the Heart can lead to erratic behavior.

During the day the *shén qi* or spirit is said to be seen in the brightness of the eyes.

49

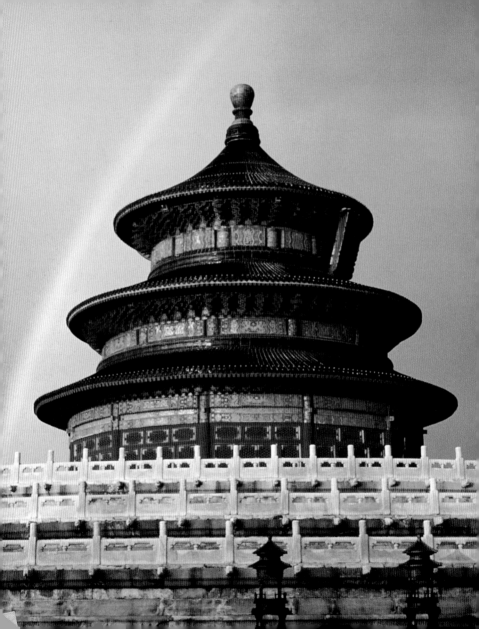

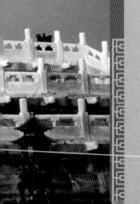

Part 2

CAUSES OF
DISEASE AND
DIAGNOSTICS

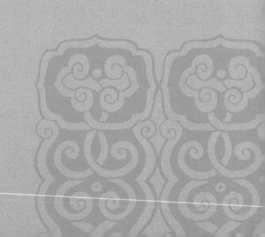

CAUSES OF DISEASE

When the theories of Chinese medicine were first formulated more than 4,000 years ago, the causes of any disease could be described only in terms of symptoms and effects. There were no machines to identify precisely what was going on in the human body, so the symptoms defined the condition.

In the *Yellow Emperor's Classic of Internal Medicine* only two causes of disease were identified: climatic factors and dysfunction of the human body. Exterior causes were labeled as *yang* while those coming from within the body were described as *yin* diseases. According to the *Nei Jing*, the external disorders could be caused by rain, wind, cold, or summer heat, while the internal problems may have their roots in improper diet, irregular life, intemperate sexuality, extreme joy, or anger. Later, in around CE 300, another classic text, entitled the *Synopsis of the Golden Chamber* and written by Zhang Zhongjing, expanded this definition to include three "injuries." These could be injuries to the Channels and collateral meridians caused by pathogenic factors invading the internal organs; injury to the body surface by pathogenic factors that then enter the body and eventually obstruct the flow of Blood. Thirdly, there were injuries caused by factors such as wounds. Today these are described as "pathogenic" factors (evil *qi*) which may be "endogenous," "exogenous," or "neither endogenous or exogenous." These pathogenic factors cause disease when they upset the balance between *yin* and *yang* or *qi* and Blood—a balance sometimes called the "unity of opposites."

Zhang Zhongjing is one of China's earliest known physicians.

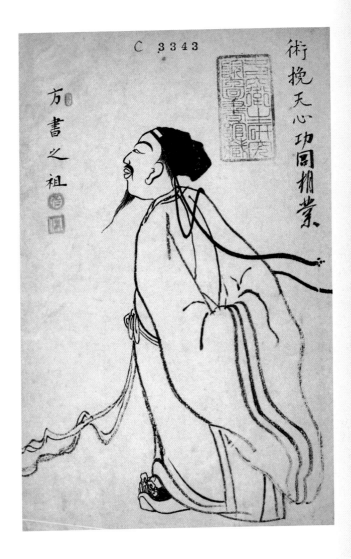

方書之祖

術挽天心功同相業

C 3343

EXTERNAL CAUSES OF DISEASE: THE SIX EVILS

To the Yellow Emperor and his contemporaries, external causes of disease were to do with the climate—seasonal disorders bringing regular and predictable illnesses. It was a view also held by the ancient Greeks and Egyptians and even now we still talk of catching a cold rather than contracting a virus or infection.

Climate in central China was, and is, a matter of extremes: freezing winters, sweltering summers, and, at times, persistent winds blowing across the Asian steppes. Small wonder then that the exogenous pathogenic factors, known as the six evils (*liù yīn*) were defined as:

- Wind (*fēng*)
- Cold (*hán*)
- Heat (*rè*)
- Dampness (*shī*)
- Dryness (*zào*)
- Fire (*huǒ*)

Wind, Heat, Fire, and Dryness are all regarded as *yang* evils while Cold and Damp are classified as *yin*.

While these evils can bring disease they are also essential to life: no wet season and there are no crops, no summer sun and crops will not ripen. However, if the six evils become excessive or abnormally extreme or if the body is weakened then these exogenous pathogens will upset the body's inner balance leading to ill health. Typically, disease is not caused by a single pathogenic factor but by a combination such as Wind-Heat or Cold-Damp. The external pathogens invade the body from the exterior via the skin, mouth, or nose and, if not

Icy winters were seen as a cause of disease with too much Cold leading to ill health.

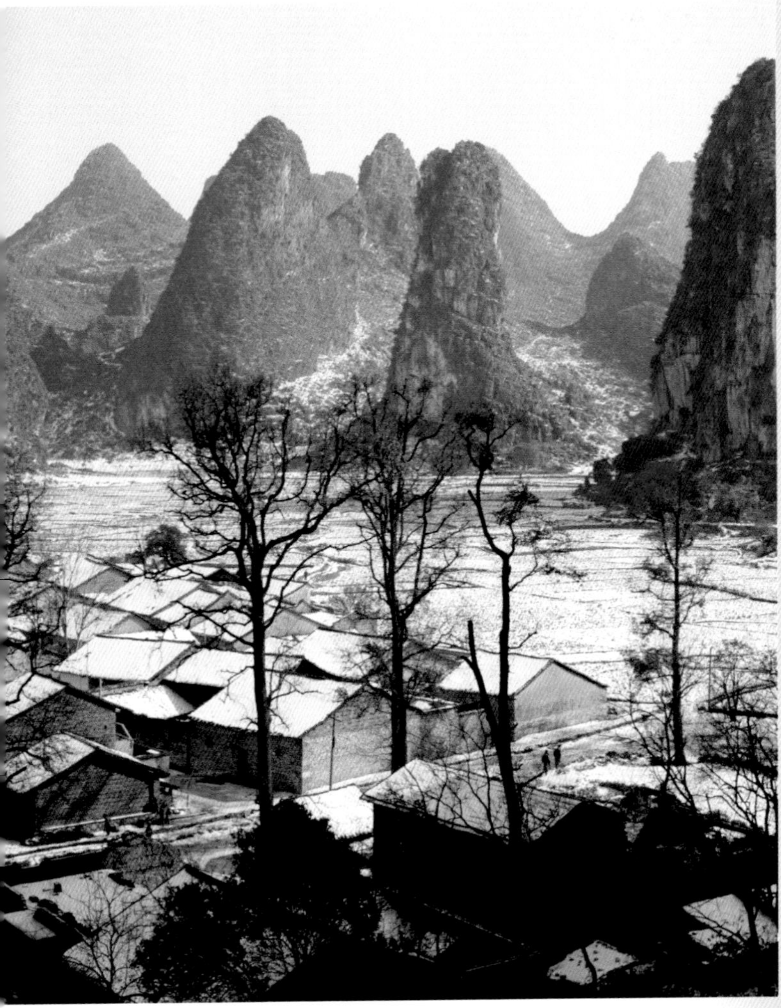

treated at that stage, can go on to affect internal organs.

Occasionally, the six evils can also originate from within the body due to organ dysfunction, but the effects are generally regarded as similar to external attack.

WIND

Although Wind (*fēng*) is associated with spring, pathogenic Wind problems can occur at any time of year. Wind is *yang* in nature, moving outward and upward and tends to attack *yang* parts of the body, notably the surface and upper parts including head, upper torso, and limbs. Since it attacks the body surface, sweating is often a symptom.

Wind disorders tend to have sudden onset and are characterized by rapid change with variable symptoms. Rheumatism, for example, is seen as a Wind disease with aches and pains often occurring in several different places.

Allergic rashes are Wind-related, as are strokes and facial paralysis. Wind can also occur in constant movement so diseases that involve abnormal motion—such as dizziness, tremors, convulsions, or unusual spasms—are also linked to Wind. The Liver is believed to be especially sensitive to attack by pathogenic Wind.

SYMPTOMS AND DISORDERS ASSOCIATED WITH WIND

Exogenous Wind is the cause of typical common colds with fever, sweating, sore throat, cough, catarrh, and aversion to wind.

Wind–Cold leads to an intolerance of both wind and cold with fever, headache, or more general aches and pains, nasal catarrh, and cough. Unlike exogenous Wind in this form of attack there is no sweating.

Wind–Heat symptoms include fever, sweating, headache, reddened eyes, sore throat, sensitivity to light, thirst, cough with thick yellow sputum, breathing problems, constipation, and possible nose bleeds or blood streaked sputum.

Wind-Dampness is much like a common cold but with pain in the limbs, lethargy, nausea, loss of appetite, and diarrhea, or as arthritis with pain shifting between various joints and muscles, which is often affected by changes in the weather.

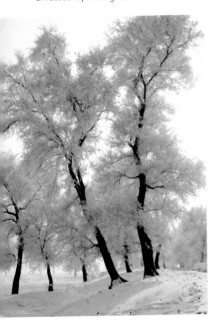

Endogenous Wind attacks the Liver leading to dizziness, muscle spasms, convulsions, and sudden coma.

COLD

Cold (*hán*) is associated with winter and is characterized by the same phenomena associated with the season: lack of motion, freezing, or coagulation. Cold is a *yin* pathogen and inhibits *yang qi* suppressing defensive energies. If it enters the body Cold tends to affect the Spleen and Stomach upsetting the normal distribution of nutrients and water.

Cold diseases are generally accompanied by pain as they can disrupt the normal smooth flow of *qi*, Blood, and body fluids with stagnation. If Cold attacks the body surface then headaches and generalized aches and pains follow; if it attacks the interior then abdominal pains are more characteristic.

Cold diseases are associated with pain as cold is still and causes stagnation.

Like freezing water, Cold causes contraction closing the pores of the skin and tightening muscles thus affecting the circulation of *yang qi* with muscle spasms and cramps that may affect the limbs or abdomen. Cold particularly affects the Kidney leading to lower back pain.

SYMPTOMS AND DISORDERS ASSOCIATED WITH COLD

Superficial Exogenous Cold is typified by intolerance to cold, fever without sweating, pains in the neck, aching joints, cough, and breathing problems.

Interior Exogenous Cold occurs when Cold injures the Stomach and Spleen or impairs Kidney *yang*— symptoms include aversion to cold, shivering, numbness, high facial color, and purple lips, diarrhea, flatulence, abdominal pain relieved by heat, poor appetite, vomiting, and muscle rigidity.

Wind–Cold–Dampness with predominant Cold is a form of arthritis with Wind-Cold-Damp in the channels and joints that can be relieved by heat and is worse in cold weather.

Endogenous Cold is when both *yang* and *qi* are deficient and symptoms include intolerance of cold, cold hands and feet, vomiting with clear fluid, watery stools, excessive urination, lethargy, and tiredness with some localized pain.

HEAT

Pathogenic Heat (*rè*) is closely associated with climate and appears only in hot summers. It leads to an excess of *yang qi*, which results in high fever, thirst and sweating, and also decreases body fluids with excessive sweating and *qi* Deficiency. Heat disorders often occur with pathogenic Dampness associated with summer's increase in humidity.

SYMPTOMS AND DISORDERS ASSOCIATED WITH HEAT

Exposure to Summer Heat: this is generally a mild condition which

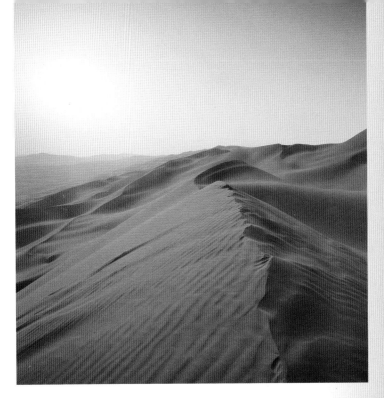

includes thirst, dry lips, sweating, possible feverishness, headache, lethargy, nausea, and dizziness.

Heat Stroke is a more severe progression of exposure to Summer Heat with increased giddiness, nausea, fever, sweating, and restlessness; in the most severe cases there may be coma and cold limbs.

The excess heat of high summer can combine with humidity to cause Damp–Heat syndromes.

Damp–Heat when combined with Damp, pathogenic Heat gives rise to spells of chills and fever, restlessness, thirst, nausea, breathing problems, poor appetite, lethargy, loose stools, and reduced urination.

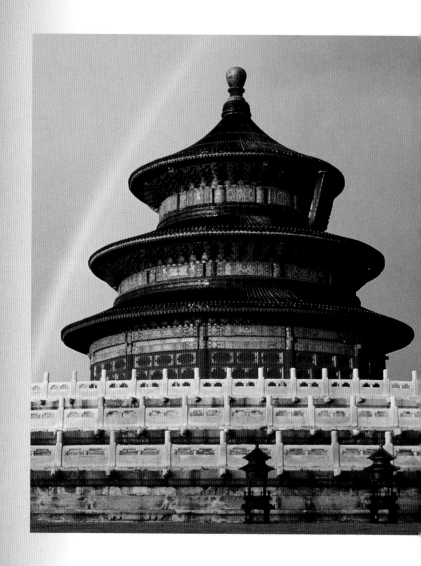

DAMPNESS

In Chinese medicine, Dampness (*shī*) is associated with late summer, a time of high humidity. However, pathogenic Damp is also linked to wet, rainy weather and can be a problem for those living in damp places, wearing wet clothing, or working with water. Damp can also originate inside the body, usually from Spleen dysfunction leading to water retention.

Damp, like Cold, is a *yin* factor so can damage the normal flow of *qi* and affect *yang*, notably Spleen *yang*. Dampness is also perceived as heavy and turbid so has a downward motion with swelling in the legs or feelings of sluggishness. It also creates sticky, turbid secretions, such as mucus in the stools, cloudy urine, vaginal discharge, sticky eyes, or weeping eczema.

Pathogenic Dampness can be caused both by excess humidity and seasonal rains and wet weather.

While problems associated with other external evils can lead to minor self-limiting conditions, such as the common cold, those associated with Damp can be difficult to clear. This is because the nature of Damp is stagnant and diffuse so Damp illnesses tend to spread, recur, and prove particularly intransigent. Stagnation can create a feeling of fullness in the Large Intestine as well as excess phlegm, profuse sputum, vomiting, and pain in the joints.

SYMPTOMS AND DISORDERS ASSOCIATED WITH DAMPNESS

Exogenous Dampness affects the normal flow of *qi* leading to vomiting, nausea and feelings of oppression in the chest and upper abdomen. There can also be poor appetite, reduced urination, and constipation. Exogenous Dampness can also cause arthritic pains with heaviness in the joints and difficulties in moving.

Wind–Dampness with predominant Dampness is associated with both the common cold and arthritis, and the condition is more likely to manifest as low fever, lethargy, and pain in the limbs.

Endogenous Dampness is generally associated with fluid retention due to Deficient Spleen with symptoms such as poor appetite, nausea, lack of thirst, a feeling of fullness in the abdomen and head, lethargy, diarrhea, edema, and, in women, abnormal vaginal discharge.

DRYNESS

Dryness (*zào*) in Chinese theory is associated with autumn when leaves dry out and turn brown. Pathogenic Dryness is a *yang* factor that depletes body fluids causing dryness in the mouth, nose and throat as well as dry, chapped skin, constipation, and reduced urine. Typically, Dryness attacks the Lung and Kidney as well as their related *fu* organs, the Large Intestine and Urinary Bladder. Kidney *yin* is important in developing body fluids and is depleted by pathogenic Dryness leading to deficiency.

Equally, Kidney or Lung weakness can reduce fluid production and result in Endogenous Dryness.

SYMPTOMS AND DISORDERS ASSOCIATED WITH DRYNESS
Exogenous Dryness (warm) is associated with hot weather with symptoms including fever, dry cough, aversion to cold, headache, and restlessness.

Exogenous Dryness (cool) is more associated with Dryness in the cool autumn and is similarly typified by fever, an aversion to cold, headache, and dry cough as well as an absence of sweating, blocked nose, and dry mouth and throat.

Endogenous Dryness is sometimes called "insufficiency of Fluids" or "Dryness of Blood" and results in dry mouth and throat, dry, rough skin, dull hair, reduced urine, dry stools, and weight loss.

The brown leaves of autumn typify the concept of pathogenic Dryness which can cause fevers.

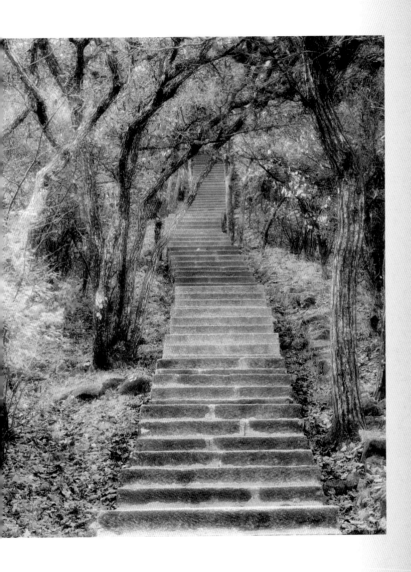

FIRE

Fire (*huǒ*) can occur at any time of the year and is a *yang* pathogen mainly affecting the head since Fire's motion is rapidly upward. Fire in the Heart, for example, which is linked to the tongue, tends to produce ulcers and soreness in that part of the mouth. Fire in the Liver is associated with sore, red eyes. Fire is also drying so symptoms are likely to include thirst, constipation, concentrated urine, and dry mouth.

Fire problems can also damage body fluids and can lead to "Fire stirring up Wind," a condition that generally affects the Liver Channel and can lead to coma, high fever, and delirium. Fire also increases the flow of Blood, which can damage the blood vessels and lead to various forms of bleeding, from nose bleeds, and blood in the urine to internal hemorrhages. Internal or endogenous Fire can be caused by a disharmony between *yin* and *yang*, which can lead either to Excess *yang* or Deficient *yin*.

Chinese theory also maintains that pathogenic Fire can be created by an excess of any of the other five evils as well as the seven emotions, the main causes of internal illness (see pages 66–71).

SYMPTOMS AND DISORDERS ASSOCIATED WITH FIRE

Exogenous Fire is associated with infectious diseases and high fever, sweating, thirst, intolerance of heat, preference for cold drinks, and, in severe cases, delirium, unconsciousness and bleeding (due to fire stirring up Endogenous Wind).

Endogenous Fire (Excess *yang*) may cause Heart, Liver, Lung, and Stomach to be affected with typical symptoms including mouth ulcers, pink eyes, a bitter taste in the mouth, anxiety, dry and sore throat, yellow sputum, painful gums, thirst, constipation, and strongly concentrated urine.

Endogenous Fire (Deficient *yin*) may cause Lung, Kidney, Heart, and

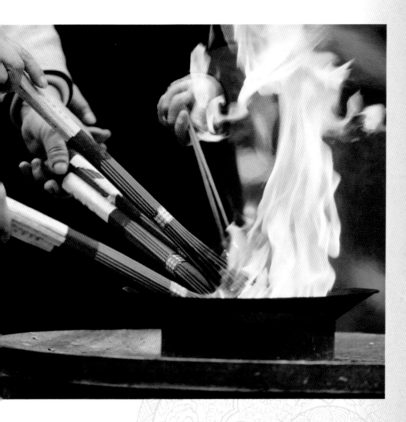

Liver to be affected with typical symptoms including insomnia and night sweats, a hot sensation on the palms of the hand or soles of the feet, dry throat and eyes, dizziness, and ringing in the ears.

Fire's motion is upward so Fire-related symptoms can often affect the head, eyes, and mouth.

INTERNAL CAUSES OF DISEASE: SEVEN EMOTIONS

In traditional Chinese theory, internal disease is believed to be produced by emotional upsets, caused by seven emotions (*qi qíng*). Each of the five *zang* organs is associated with a particular emotion and any imbalance in this emotion—excess or deficiency—can lead to dysfunction of the relevant organ.

In everyday life emotions are seen as the normal reaction to external events, and it is only when these emotions become extreme or are missing altogether, that they are seen as pathogenic factors.

Although there are only five organs, there are seven defined emotions with two associated with both Heart and Lung:

- Joy (*xī*)
- Anger (*nù*)
- Sadness (*bēi*)
- Worry (*sī*)
- Fear (*kŏng*)
- Grief (*yōu*)
- Shock or Fright (*jīng*)

The Heart plays a pivotal role in emotional disorders as it is said to house consciousness and govern all the *zang-fu* organs so emotional stimuli are believed to attack the Heart first before moving on to the relevant organ.

The different emotions are also believed to disrupt the normal flow of *qi*. According to the *Yellow Emperor's Classic of Internal Medicine* (*Nei Jing*) Anger causes *qi* to flow upward while Fear causes it to descend and Worry leads to *qi* stagnation. Both the Heart and Liver are especially susceptible to emotional disorders.

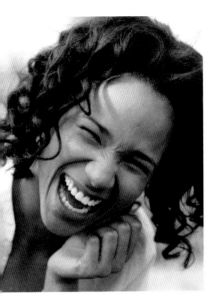

Excessive Joy is seen as a negative emotion which can damage Heart *qi.*

ordered society very different to our own. In today's world the noisy, excited behavior of teenagers shouting together in the street, for example, would be seen as negative aspects of Joy likely to damage the Heart and also possibly affect the Lung. Excess Joy is said to scatter Heart *qi* leading to an inability to concentrate. The sort of hysterical laughter associated with some forms of mental disorder is also associated by the Chinese with damaged Heart *qi.*

JOY

Joy (*xī*) is the emotion associated with the Heart; it encourages the circulation of *qi* and Blood and is seen as a beneficial emotion. However, Excess Joy, in Chinese theory, is seen as over-exuberance verging on mania.

One has to remember that these theories evolved in a hierarchical,

ANGER

The emotion associated with the Liver is anger (*nù*) and an excess can affect the flow of Liver *qi*, which interrupts over-all circulation of *qi* and Blood. It can also lead to *qi* stagnation while the ascending Liver *qi* can interfere with normal Lung *qi* action causing disharmonies here as well.

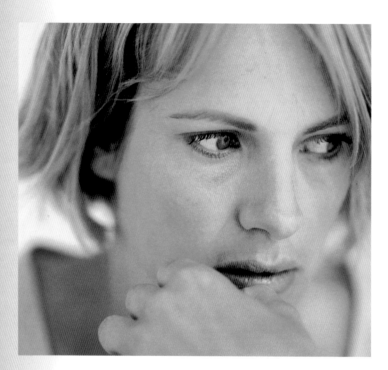

Typical symptoms of this disruptive, ascendant Liver *qi* include irritability, headaches, dizziness, flushed face, red eyes, and a bitter taste in the mouth. There may also be dryness in the throat or a sensation of something stuck in the throat, pains in the ribs, and feelings of suffocation and depression.

Worry is the emotion associated with the Spleen.

In women, anger can be related to menstrual irregularities and breast lumps; normalizing Liver *qi* is an important approach in treating various gynecological problems such as premenstrual syndrome. In extreme cases the disruption of normal Blood and *qi* flow can lead to unconsciousness or choking if Lung *qi* is severely affected.

SADNESS

Sadness (*bēi*) is linked to the Lung with excessive melancholy interrupting normal flow of Lung *qi,* causing stagnation with feelings of oppression in the chest and depression.

If Lung *qi* becomes stagnant for a long time it can lead to Fire, which affects the vital essence of the Lung, which in turn can harm the Spleen disturbing digestive function with loss of appetite, insomnia, and weight loss.

WORRY

Worry (*sī*) is associated with the Spleen, the prime *zang* organ involved in digestion so any damage to Spleen *qi* can cause problems with distributing nutrients and water to the body. While the emotion linked to the Spleen can be translated as worry, it is also sometimes referred to as pensiveness or over-thinking.

The Chinese say that pensiveness originates from the Heart and occupies one's hearing and makes one's mind concentrate. Prolonged over-thinking can thus also lead to Stagnation of Heart *qi* with symptoms of Heart disease such as strong palpitations, anxiety, weakness in the limbs, disturbed sleep, forgetfulness, and in severe cases, dementia. Some types of menstrual irregularities can also be associated with this type of *qi* Stagnation.

Prolonged Stagnation of Heart and Spleen *qi* leads to a syndrome called "Depressed Heat in the Heart and Spleen," with symptoms such as loss of appetite, constipation, mouth ulcers, insomnia, palpitations, anxiety, and a tendency to be easily startled.

FEAR

Perhaps not surprisingly, Fear (*kŏng*) is linked to the Kidney; almost all of us have a tendency for increased frequency of urination when we are frightened or nervous.

Fear differs from Shock or Fright, in that Fear is said to originate from timidity within the body and is linked to reduced functionality of the internal organs whereas Shock comes from external sources.

Fear injures the Kidney by causing the normally upward flow of Kidney *qi* to reverse and descend. This leads to low back pains, increased urination, incontinence, lethargy, listlessness, weakness in the legs and feet, and a desire for solitude. In women it can cause excessively long menstrual periods and irregular menstruation. Bedwetting in children can also be explained in these terms with severe shyness, insecurity, or timidity leading to internally generated Fear, which in turn causes incontinence.

GRIEF

Like Sadness, Grief (*yōu*) is associated with the Lung. Excessive Grief damages Lung *qi* and since it controls the *qi* flow through the body, can result in more generalized *qi* stagnation with reduced functionality among all the internal organs. Symptoms can include pallor, breathing problems, a sensation of suffocation in the chest, lethargy, depression, loss of appetite, constipation and difficulty with urination, and frequent sighing.

Breathing problems and conditions such as bronchial asthma are commonly seen in the recently bereaved.

SHOCK OR FRIGHT

Shock (*jīng*) is due to external factors rather than internal and is more like a state of panic than an internal nagging fear. It is associated with the Heart and leads to a general dysfunction of *qi*, with the

Heart *qi* said to "wander about, adhering to nothing." Symptoms include palpitations that may be strong and continual, mental restlessness, cold sweats, and a tendency to be easily startled—the sort of symptoms which in the West we might label a "panic attack." Unexplained crying or upsets in babies and infants are often attributed to Fright.

Grief can lead to such disorders as bronchial asthma.

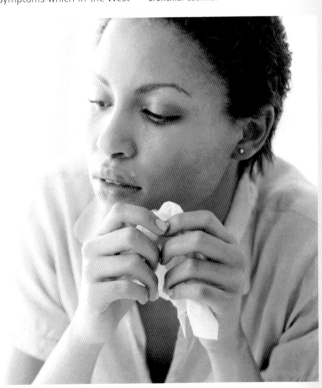

OTHER CAUSES OF DISEASE

Chinese traditional medicine also defines a range of other causes of disease that are neither external/climatic nor internal/emotional. Some practitioners prefer to classify these various causes as additional external or internal factors. The pseudo-external causes are: pestilence and traumatic injuries, insect or animal bites, and parasitic infestation, while the internal-like conditions include: irregular diet, excess sexual activity and physical exertion, excess Phlegm, and Blood Stasis. In addition there are congenital causes.

TRAUMATIC INJURIES, BITES AND PARASITIC INFESTATIONS

This group of diseases is usually dealt with by modern surgery and antibiotics. In bygone ages they could, in severe cases, lead to massive infections, poorly healed wounds, hemorrhages, or death. Today, they are the sorts of incidents that see sufferers heading for the nearest accident and emergency department.

Parasitic infestations are slightly different since many can go undetected for some time, while others do not always respond to antibiotics or other modern medicines. Typical symptoms of the various pinworms, nematodes, hookworms, tapeworms, or flukes that can infect our guts include abdominal pains, itching, and sallow complexion. The classic Chinese diagnosis in such cases is "Acute abdominal pain with cold limbs due to worms." Schistosomes (Bilharzia) is a type of fluke found mainly in tropical areas that causes serious illness and is rather differently described as "disturbing Blood circulation leading to Stagnant Blood and retention of Water in the abdomen."

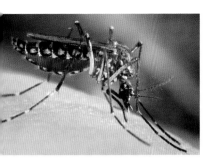

Biting insects and parasites are a significant cause of disease in hot countries.

PESTILENCE

This category basically covers the range of epidemic infections caused by viruses and bacteria, which is now largely controlled by antibiotics and mass vaccinations. In an earlier age, these illnesses were of unknown origin, with sudden onset, acute symptoms, and frequent fatalities.

IRREGULAR DIET

Sometimes defined as an internal cause of disease, irregular diet is seen as an important pathogenic factor. It can injure Spleen and Stomach by disturbing the normal pattern of processing and distributing nutrients and water through the body leading to disruption in the flow of *qi*, Blood, and body fluids. With these normal flows disrupted there can be a build-up in Damp leading to the production of Phlegm and symptoms of endogenous Heat. Over time these disruptions can affect other organs causing serious illness. In Chinese theory irregular diet can have three distinct causes: volume, improper food, and rotten or infected food.

VOLUME OF FOOD

Food should be taken in the right amount at the right time and both excess food or eating too little can lead to disease. Too little food means there are insufficient nutrients to transform into *qi* and Blood, resulting in weakness in vital energy and weakened *wèi qi*, causing a likely increase in external illness. Too much food damages Spleen and Stomach leading to abdominal distention, belching, foul-smelling stools, and an accumulation of undigested food that is transformed into Heat and

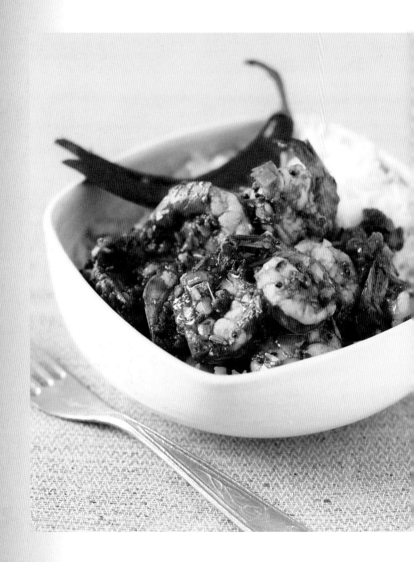

may produce Phlegm. Traditionally, meals are eaten at 6 am, 12 noon, and 6 pm, which are believed to be the correct intervals between meals for ideal digestion.

IMPROPER FOOD

This may be due to an imbalance in what is available locally, such as the traditional shortage of fruits in winter, or could be associated with personal preference and the avoidance of certain food groups. Either factor can lead to disorders such as goiter, rickets, night blindness, and beriberi.

Personal preferences are also significant. Too much raw or cold food, for example, is said to lead to Spleen and Stomach Deficiency, with abdominal pains and diarrhea. Too much spicy or pungent food, in contrast, impairs the vital essence of the Stomach, leading to a condition called "Excess Stomach Heat."

Food needs to be balanced to prevent disharmony—"cold" prawns with "hot" chillies, for example.

with feelings of hunger, indigestion, vertigo, and possibly ulcers and boils.

Too much alcohol is believed to cause an increase in Damp, Heat, and Phlegm, with ancient texts describing the resulting abdominal masses and weight loss in much the same terms that a modern physician would define cirrhosis.

ROTTEN OR INFECTED FOOD

Eating bad food causes what most people would call food poisoning, with nausea, vomiting, diarrhea, abdominal pain, or dysentery.

EXCESS SEXUAL ACTIVITY AND PHYSICAL EXERTION

Sometimes classified as another internal cause of disease, too much sexual activity is believed to consume _jīng_ and damage Kidney _qi_ leading to Deficiency with lower back pains, aching knee joints, dizziness, tinnitus, and lethargy. In men there may be impotence and

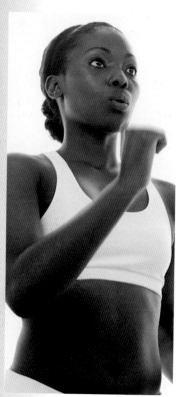

In Chinese medicine an excess of energetic exercise is seen as harmful.

leading to reduced functionality in all the *zang-fu* organs, with general sluggishness, lethargy, apathy, and breathing disorders. Like excess Worry or over-thinking, excess physical activity can also affect Heart *qi* with resulting palpitations, insomnia, forgetfulness, and disturbed sleep. Too little physical exertion can be just as damaging, with a deficiency in vital energy and reduced *wèi qi* since the circulation of both *qi* and Blood will be slow. Symptoms include poor appetite, lethargy, generalized weakness in the limbs, vertigo, and palpitations.

EXCESS PHLEGM

Phlegm in Chinese medicine is quite different from the "phlegm" that Western medicine associates with catarrhal conditions and sputum. Phlegm, in this context, is believed to develop from Water and Fluid retained in the body. Phlegm can be

nocturnal emissions while women typically suffer from menstrual irregularities and vaginal discharge.

In contrast, too much physical exertion weakens primordial *qi*

visible or invisible: the visible appears as sputum but the invisible collects inside the body and can be the cause of disease and its result.

In Chinese theory the Spleen separates the clear and turbid fluids produced during digestion. If these turbid fluids are not excreted but retained because of some failure in the water transport system, then they can develop into Phlegm. This failure can be due to *qi* weakness in Lung, Spleen, or Kidney or may be associated with obstructions in the Triple Burner (*san jiao*) disrupting the normal Fluid transport mechanisms.

Pathogenic (invisible) Phlegm can collect anywhere in the body, in any of the *zang-fu* organs or in superficial tissues such as tendons and skin. There may be visible external signs of Phlegm, such as edema, oozing fluid from inflammations, or palpable lymph nodes. Internal symptoms can include mental disturbances, blockages in the Channels, or

accumulations of Phlegm in specific organs. If Phlegm builds up in the Heart, for example, there will be mental disturbances, such as schizophrenia or mania while Phlegm in the Lungs can cause asthmatic symptoms or productive coughs with characteristics wheezy breathing described as "the sound of Phlegm."

Stagnation in the Stomach can cause nausea and vomiting, while in the Channels it can lead to sensations of numbness and partial paralysis.

BLOOD STASIS

Blood Stagnation or Stasis is another of the possible internal causes of disease. Blood, in Chinese medicine, is not the same as our usual anatomical concept of blood and Blood Stagnation does not imply a thrombosis or massive clot somewhere in the circulatory system.

Stagnant Blood is a pathological product caused when organs fail to work properly; Stasis occurs when

Blood flows erratically because of *qi* Deficiency or because of attack by pathogenic Cold. Internal bleeding caused either by trauma or pathogenic Heat can also lead to Blood Stasis. Stagnant Blood can also cause an obstruction and further interrupt the flow of *qi* and Blood. Once Stasis has developed, the Blood involved is no longer free to circulate in the body moistening the tissues and nourishing the body so causing further problems.

Typical symptoms of Blood Stasis vary depending on whereabouts in the body it is stagnating but generally include some sort of pain and swelling. Stagnation in the Lungs, for example, causes chest pain and coughing up blood; in the Liver it can lead to pain and abdominal masses; in the Stomach to obvious bright red blood in the stools.

Stagnant Blood in the uterus is the cause of many menstrual problems, including period pain, irregular menstruation, and absence of periods.

CONGENITAL CONDITIONS

The final cause of illness in Chinese theory is congenital—problems we are born with. Both primordial *qi* and congenital *jīng* are derived from our parents and there is little we can do if these are weak and insufficient. Damage to the fetus or birth defects are similarly seen as beyond our control—although in parts of China it is still common to give babies an herbal brew at 15 days old, designed to clear the Heat and Toxins that are believed to be present at birth.

Both premature birth and the mother's state of health during pregnancy are also seen as congenital influences on future health and, although it is possible to support congenital *qi* and *jīng* by strengthening grain *qi* and air *qi* and post-natal *jīng* with healthy diet and lifestyle, overcoming congenital weaknesses remains challenging.

In Chinese theory much of our vital energy is derived from our parents.

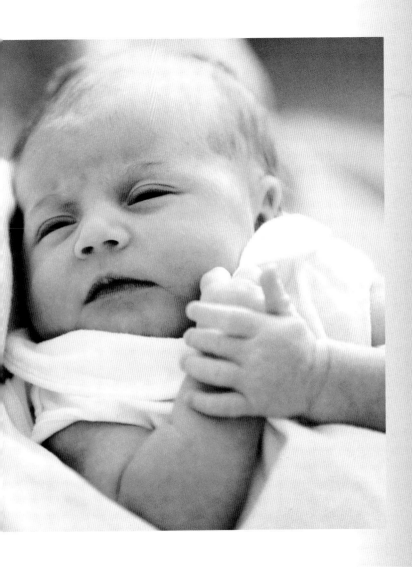

THE DEVELOPMENT OF DISEASE

While Chinese theory has clearly defined causes of disease, the progression and outcome are not as certain since much depends on the strength of the body to fight back and overcome the illness. It is a contest between the pathogen and what some call anti-pathogenic *qi*.

ANTI-PATHOGENIC *QI*

Fighting illness, in Chinese theory, is about balance: about adjusting the interaction between *yin* and *yang*, between *qi* and Blood and between the various functions of the *zang-fu* organs in order to defeat the invading pathogen.

It is also about prevention: as Zhang Zhongjing put it in the *Synopsis of the Golden Chamber*: "Keep strong and disease will find no way to attack."

Four main factors are believed to determine the strength of each individual's anti-pathogenic *qi*:

Constitution which is largely dictated by the attributes inherited from our parents plus the influences of lifestyle and environment which follow.

Diet which is important among the "after heaven" influences with both obesity and low body weight affecting how we combat disease.

Mental state which in traditional Chinese medicine has significant influence on the function of *qi* and Blood. Depression, for example, can lead to poor appetite, organ dysfunction, and weakened *wèi qi* making the sufferer more susceptible to pathogenic attack.

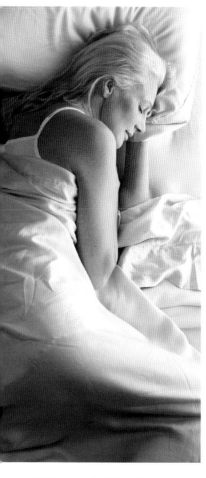

Excessive sleep in Chinese theory is believed to weaken *qi*.

Poor habits Poor habits which generally involve excess: excessive sleeping, for example, weakens *qi*; too much sitting harms muscles; too much standing—bones; or too much walking—tendons; while excessive concentration on mental work for long hours injures Heart and Spleen.

Recovery from illness means that anti-pathogenic *qi* has won the battle; deterioration in the condition obviously means the reverse. In Chinese theory most illnesses start from exterior symptoms that move to the interior if the condition worsens. The second stage is the development of Cold symptoms as defeat of anti-pathogenic *qi* damages the body's Heat. Finally, Deficiency symptoms develop as anti-pathogenic *qi* weakens even further with, ultimately, life ending when "*yin* and *yang* part and *qi* and Blood run out." Good treatment is focused on preventing the illness moving through these states.

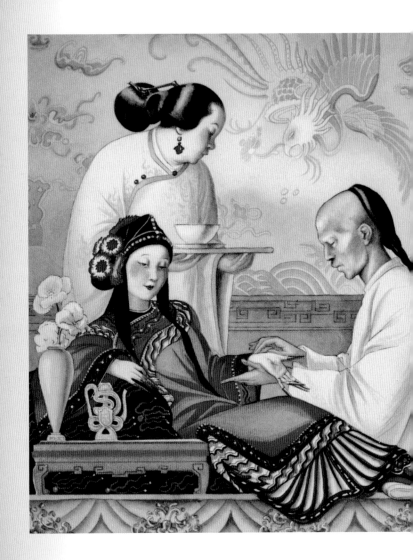

RESTORING BALANCE

Recovery from illness means that the anti-pathogenic *qi* has successfully re-balanced *yin* and *yang*, *qi* and Blood, as well as normalizing the various functions of the *zang-fu* organs. Medical treatment is aimed at identifying the various imbalances and supporting the action of the anti-pathogenic *qi* at each stage.

Vital energy (*yang qi*) and vital essence (*yin* essence) are constantly changing with vital energy producing Heat and motion upward while vital essence is associated with Cold and tranquillity moving downward. Imbalance occurs when there is failure of either vital energy or vital essence.

Similarly, *qi* and Blood are mutually interdependent with Blood being the material basis for generating *qi* and the flow of Blood depending on *qi*.

Chinese physicians monitor signs and symptoms closely to assess the disease progression.

Any weakness in *qi* can lead to a reduction in that flow and thus stagnation of Blood, while a weakness in Blood interrupts the generation of *qi*.

Each of the *zang-fu* organs is either involved in some form of ascending or descending motion. In illness these natural movements can be disrupted causing a range of symptoms that the Chinese physician will use to identify the precise organ weaknesses involved.

There are five ways that *yang* and *yin* can be disrupted, four interruptions for normal *qi* and Blood function and a great many symptoms that result from interrupting the normal ascending and descending functions of the *zang-fu* organs.

YANG DISRUPTION

Dominant *yang* is usually caused by pathogenic Heat attacking the body or by pathogenic Cold entering the body and being transformed into Heat.

Deficient *yang* is usually from innate insufficiency or after a long illness.

Perished *yang* is a serious condition where *yang* becomes detached from the body either because of severe deficiency or extreme Cold.

Excessive *yang* **hindering** *yin* occurs when dominant *yang* produces excess Heat in the interior that becomes disconnected with *yin* on the exterior.

Impaired *yang* **impeding the creation of** *yin* occurs when persistent deficiency of *yang* reduces the vital essence.

YIN DISRUPTION
Dominant *yin* is usually caused by Cold and Damp attacking the exterior and a failure of the *yang qi* to produce warmth.

Deficient *yin* is generally due to excessive consumption of vital essence, possibly related to fever.

Perished *yin* is usually due to excess Heat scorching body fluids but also

caused by massive hemorrhage, severe diarrhea or vomiting, and generally signifying a critical condition.

Excessive *yin* **hindering** *yang* occurs when too much *yin* creates excess Cold that is trapped within the body and *yang* becomes separated on the exterior.

Impaired *yin* **impeding the creation of** *yang* is caused by over-consumption of vital essence damaging the production of vital energy with, ultimately, a deficiency of both.

INTERRUPTED QI FUNCTION
Deficient *qi* is primarily due to malfunction of Spleen, Kidney or possibly Lung.

Stagnant *qi* is usually due to obstruction caused when the *zang-fu* organs fail to manage the normal ascending and descending processes. It is most commonly found in depression when there is stagnation of Phlegm or Dampness.

Qi sinking to the middle *jiao* is a variant of *qi* deficiency linked to a failure of *qi* to ascend with weakness of Spleen *qi*.

Adverse flow of *qi* is usually an abnormal upward flow of *qi* from the Lung, Liver, Stomach or *chong* Channel related to impaired emotions or excessive consumption of cold food.

INTERRUPTED BLOOD FUNCTION

Deficient Blood may be due to massive hemorrhage, a failure of the Spleen and Stomach to transform food and water correctly, or internal damage due to chronic illness or parasites.

Stagnant Blood is usually where the circulation is damaged by pathogenic factors, traumatic injury, or weakened *qi*. In women it can be caused by retention of the lochia after childbirth.

Blood attacked by Heat is when both exogenous and endogenous Heat can damage Blood or external Cold can invade the interior and be transformed into Heat. Emotional depression can also cause Heat by depressing Liver *qi* leading to internal Fire.

Hemorrhage is believed to be caused by an adverse flow of *qi*, external injury or excess Fire.

FAILURE OF ASCENDING AND DESCENDING MOTIONS

Numerous conditions can follow from a failure of the normal motions associated with the *zang-fu* organs. If Lung *qi* fails to descend, for example, there can be coughing and asthmatic problems, while over-exuberant Liver *qi* has an upward motion causing dizziness and headaches. If the downward motion associated with the Large Intestine fails, constipation is likely, while weakness in the Spleen can cause *qi* to descend and so fail to support surrounding tissues with the risk of rectal or uterine prolapse.

CHINESE EXAMINATION

Dating back to an age when doctors depended on what they could see, feel, and hear rather than a battery of clinical tests, traditional Chinese examination follows an established pattern based on observation and listening. There are four distinct phases to a traditional Chinese examination: inspection; auscultation and olfaction; interrogation; and palpation.

INSPECTION

Inspection is the most important component of the examination and involves studying the patient's appearance, tongue, nose, skin color, and so on. A physician will start the examination from the moment they see the patient: how do they walk or stand? What does that imply about their Spirit—is it alert and lively or dull and downcast? If the body is firm and muscular then *qi* and *jīng* are likely to be strong and the person healthy; obesity can suggest Spleen *qi* Deficiency with failure to transform nutrients or possibly a Phlegm or Damp problem. The

extremely thin could be suffering from digestive weakness, perhaps middle *jiao* problems or maybe *yin* Deficiency.

The over-active and restless might be suffering from a *yang* syndrome, Excess or Heat while the more passive could have a *yin* imbalance, Deficiency or Cold. Tremors are also significant: in the elderly, trembling hands imply *yin* deficiency, while in younger people this is more likely to be related to a Wind problem.

The colors and shapes seen in the eyes, face, and tongue also each have their own specific significance.

INSPECTING THE EYES

The eyes are said to be the "door of the Spirit" and a physician will look for any signs of swelling or discoloration. If the Spirit is strong and alert then the eyes are bright and shining; if not they can look dull and blank or glassy—both of which suggest weakened spirit. Different parts of the eye correspond to different organs so a yellow discharge in the corner of the eye may suggest some sort of problem with Heat in the Heart while swollen eyelids can imply Spleen weakness. Color is important, too: red eyes suggest some form of Heat problem while if the whites of the eyes (the sclera) have a yellowish tinge it suggests Damp.

THE EYE

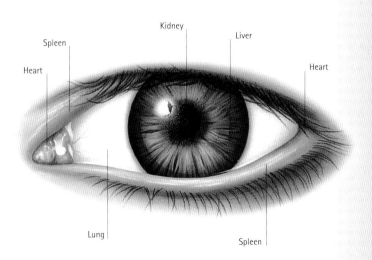

Kidney

Liver

Spleen

Heart

Heart

Lung

Spleen

INSPECTING THE FACE

The color of the face is also significant in diagnosis: if it is very red or flushed, there may be excess Heat or if the flushing only appears in the evening *yin* Deficiency is likely. If it is white or very pale then the opposite is true with a likely Cold syndrome or possible *yang* or *qi* Deficiency. Yellow suggests Damp or Spleen problems while greenish tinges imply Cold or Blood Stagnation.

The location of any unusual colors, inflammations or sores around the nose and cheeks is also indicative of underlying disorders in the *zang-fu* organs. Redness between nose and lip, for example, suggests a uterine problem in women while the areas beneath the eyes are associated with the Kidney.

Different parts of the body are also related through the five-element model to the *zang-fu* organs so the quality of the head hair can provide insights about the Kidney, while abnormally pale lips

THE TONGUE

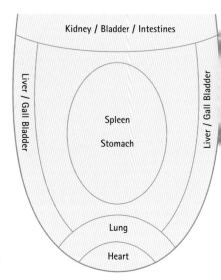

may suggest a Spleen weakness and broken weak nails some form of Liver dysfunction.

INSPECTING THE TONGUE

The tongue is another important pointer in diagnosis with different parts of the tongue relating to different organs of the body, while the color and type of coating can indicate which pathogenic

SOME OF THE POSSIBLE HEALTH PROBLEMS ASSOCIATED WITH PARTICULAR TONGUE COLORS

Pale	Cold syndrome, *yang* Deficiency, *qi* Deficiency, Blood Deficiency
Reddish	Interior Heat syndrome, Excess *qi* and Blood, *yin* Deficiency
Dark red	Severe endogenous Heat
Purple or blue	Inadequate body fluids, extreme pathogenic Heat
Purplish spots	Blood Stagnation
Black	Internal Cold syndrome
Yellow coating	Heat syndrome, Excess Damp or endogenous pathogens
White coating	Cold syndrome or exogenous pathogens
Cracked surface	Consumption of vital essence

factors are involved in the illness. A red tip, for example, could suggest Heat in the Heart while redness to the back of the tongue could imply a Kidney problem. In general a thin, pale tongue implies Deficiency of *qi* and Blood, while cracks in the tongue's surface could suggest a Blood Deficiency and apparent tooth-marks round the edges may imply a problem with Spleen *yang*.

Yellow coatings suggest Heat, Damp or endogenous pathogens, while white coatings indicate an exogenous or Cold problem. There are dozens of possible combinations of tongue color, coating, shape, blemishes, and motion and each will suggest a specific syndrome or health problem to the experienced practitioner.

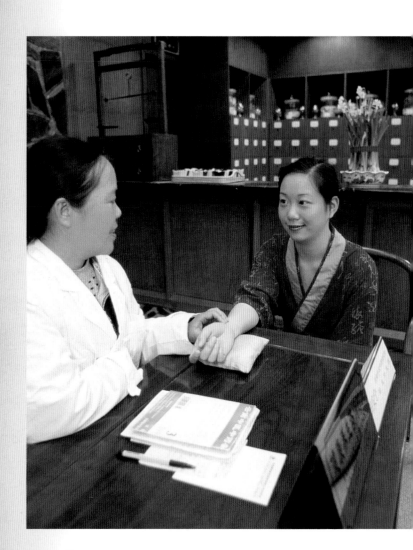

AUSCULTATION AND OLFACTION

After inspection comes the listening and smelling: what sort of voice does the patient have? Is their breathing fast or slow, regular or irregular? Are there any abnormal body smells? A loud voice suggests *yang*, Heat and Excess while a soft voice implies *yin*, Cold or Deficiency syndromes. Speech is linked to the Heart so impediments such as stammering or confused words could indicate an underlying Heart disorder.

Chinese practitioners measure breathing rates in comparison to their own rather than resorting to timers and stopwatches. Coughs and hiccoughs are also analysed; coughing with a low weak voice, for example, suggests Deficiency while loud hiccoughs imply Excess Heat. Strong body odor also suggests a general Heat problem.

There are four distinct stages to each consultation starting with inspection and ending with palpation.

INTERROGATION

In Chinese theory, the interrogation phase should cover "The Ten Questions," a routine developed over centuries that should be covered during the course of the consultation and, given the specific interpretations of the patient's reply which the Chinese doctor makes, can actually appear quite brief. These questions cover:

- the nature of any chills and fevers
- patterns of perspiration
- the location and type of any pains in the head, body, and limbs
- unusual sensations in chest and abdomen
- bowel movements and urination
- appetite
- thirst
- hearing
- previous diseases suffered by the patient and other family members
- onset and development of the present illness

Women will also be asked about their menstrual cycle or vaginal discharges while the focus in children is likely to be on infectious diseases, any frights, or recent changes in eating patterns.

The aim of The Ten Questions is to understand how the patient's chief complaint fits in with more general information about lifestyle and familial tendencies. It is a routine well understood by Chinese patients who will describe their pain, for example, as distending, stabbing, gaseous, burning, heavy, gnawing, dull, hot or "accompanied by cold" with very little prompting.

PALPATION

The final stage of the consultation is palpation or touching. As in the West this can include abdominal palpation looking for any lumps or masses as well as feeling the limbs to assess temperature or swellings.

The key difference in Chinese medicine, however, is in the importance placed on taking the

pulse or pulses. While a Western practitioner will simply feel the wrist to measure heart rate and check for irregular rhythms, the Chinese doctor will be subtly applying three fingers to each wrist.

The area where the radial artery can be felt on the wrist is known in Chinese as the *cun kou*, with the three finger-width points assessed known as *cun*, *guan* and *chi*. The *cun* position corresponds to the *taiyuan* point on the Lung meridian (see page 230) and, since all the *zang-fu* organs and Channels are said to meet in the Lung, it is believed to be the ideal place for measuring their strength.

While each position equates to one or other of the *zang-fu* organs, there are also different types of pressure applied by the doctor— gentle, firm, or hard—assessing how deeply the illness has penetrated from superficial to deep within the interior and giving a total of nine pulse positions. Each reading takes at least a minute to assess fully.

CHECKING THE PULSE

A normal healthy pulse is usually described as strong without being "solid," with regular rhythm and a firm root, and is felt by pressing deeply at the *chi* position. A Chinese doctor measures pulse by matching it with his or her own steady breathing with the normal rate said to be four or five beats per breath (at a breathing rate of about 18 breaths per minute). What is deemed normal varies between men and women and at different times of year. The female pulse is generally softer, weaker, and more rapid than a male pulse, while for both men and women the pulse may appear slightly taut in spring, more full in summer, floating in the autumn, and sinking in winter as our *yin-yang* balance changes with the seasons.

Classic Chinese texts talk of 28 different types of pulse although modern practitioners tend to focus on 17.

Floating pulse is superficial and feels weaker as more pressure is applied, and indicates an Exterior syndrome.

Deep pulse feels stronger when more pressure is applied, and indicates an Interior syndrome —a deep forceful pulse suggests

PULSE POSITIONS

	Left wrist	Right wrist
Cun	Heart/Pericardium	Lung
Guan	Liver/Gall Bladder	Spleen/Stomach
Chi	Kidney/Urinary	Bladder/Kidney/Large and Small Intestines

an Excess condition; a weak deep pulse a Deficiency syndrome.

Slow pulse with three or fewer than three beats per breath (less than 60 a minute) suggests Cold or *yang* Deficiency.

Rapid pulse with more than five beats per breath (more than 90 per minute) suggests a Heat condition.

Empty pulse describes the strength of the throb with an empty pulse presenting little force to the pressing fingers. It indicates Deficiency.

Full pulse is where the throbs are clearly perceptible even with little pressure. It suggests Excess.

Slippery pulse is said to feel smooth and flowing. It suggests Excess Heat or Phlegm.

Choppy pulse is the opposite of slippery—fine, short, and slow, it suggests Stagnant *qi* or Blood, or Blood Deficiency and is common in anemia.

Overflowing pulse feels like dashing waves that rise forcefully but suddenly decline. It suggests Excess Heat or the advanced stage of an infectious illness.

Thready pulse is a fine pulse that remains clear under heavy pressure. It can indicate Deficiency of *qi* and Blood or of both *yin* and *yang*.

Taut pulse feels like pressing a violin string. It usually suggests Liver or Gall Bladder problems or Phlegm.

Soft pulse lacks tension and is superficial, soft, and fine. It suggests Dampness or Deficiency or may occur in debility when *qi* and Blood are weak.

Tight pulse feels like a tightly stretched cord but is smaller and not so tense as a taut pulse. It can suggest Cold or pain.

Relaxed pulse is loose and appears slow even though it may be at the usual four beats per breath. It suggests pathogenic Damp.

Hasty pulse is rapid with irregular missing beats. It indicates Excess *yang* and Heat with stagnation of Blood and *qi*.

Slow, uneven pulse is slow with irregular missing beats. It indicates blockage of *qi* due to Excess *yin*, Cold, Phlegm, or Stagnant Blood.

Intermittent pulse has a normal frequency but a pattern of regular missing beats. This suggests general decline in the *zang* organs such as in severe Heat syndrome, severe pain, fever, or fright.

While obviously opposite patterns of pulse cannot occur together—a pulse cannot be rapid and slow at the same time, for example—other characteristics do commonly occur together. A floating, tight pulse could imply a superficial Cold problem while a deep rapid pulse implies interior Heat, and so on.

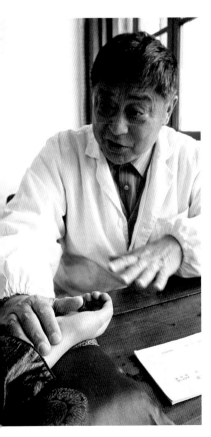

Taking the pulse is an important part of each examination, with the doctor checking on nine distinct positions.

CHINESE DIAGNOSTICS

Disease labels in Western medicine are often either descriptive of the underlying pathological problem causing the illness or of the most significant symptom: arthritis simply means inflammation of the joints; gastritis is inflammation of the stomach, and so on. It is the same with Chinese medicine, only the labels sound very different to Western ears: Deficiency of Heart *qi*, Flaring of Liver Fire, or Blood Stagnation, for example.

IDENTIFYING THE DISORDER

Identifying the correct Chinese syndrome is a far more formalized process than with Western differential diagnosis and is based on what are termed the "Eight Guiding Principles" (*ba gang*). This involves identifying whether the problem is related to Interior or Exterior, Cold or Heat, Deficiency or Excess, *yin* or *yang*. All signs and symptoms of disease, which the doctor has identified from the examination, are classified in these eight categories with a series of additional diagnostic approaches used to refine this basic differentiation and pinpoint the precise syndrome involved.

Traditionally, signs and symptoms in Chinese medicine are seen less as demonstrations of some underlying pathological condition and more as indications of how the body is fighting the invading pathogen. The same "disease" in Western terms could actually be defined as various different syndromes in Chinese medicine, reflecting how the disease is progressing in the individual patient and how the patient's body is responding depending on the individual strengths and weaknesses.

EIGHT GUIDING PRINCIPLES

First the doctor must decide whether the problem is Exterior or Interior: Exterior syndromes tend to be superficial, less severe and short-lived while Interior syndromes are more serious and often chronic. Exterior problems are usually the result of attack by one or other of the external pathogens while Interior syndromes can be associated with:

- more advanced stages of these external diseases
- direct attack on the internal *zang-fu* organs by an exogenous pathogen—by eating too much cold food, for example
- emotional disturbance related to one or other of the seven emotions

Having completed their examination Chinese physicians apply the Eight Guiding Principles to produce a diagnosis.

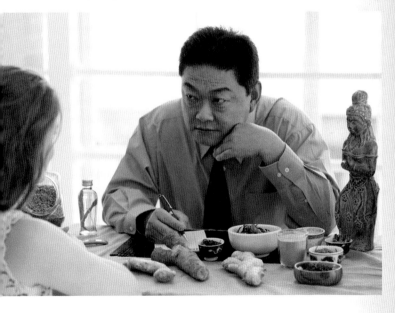

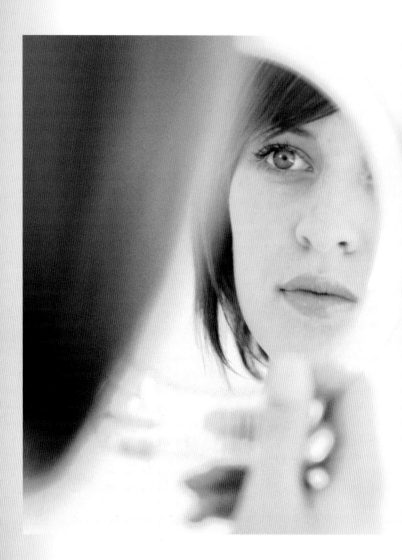

The next stage is to identify whether it is a Cold or a Heat problem. Cold syndromes may be associated with attack by pathogenic Cold or by a dominant *yin* condition associated with *yang* Deficiency, for example. Heat problems might similarly be associated with pathogenic Heat or perhaps by Fire caused by Stagnant *qi* in one of the *zang* organs.

Next comes Excess or Deficiency: Deficiency problems might be associated with weakened defense energy and thus easy success for any invading pathogens, while in Excess problems the anti-pathogenic *qi* is still strong so the struggle between the two produces symptoms of hyperactivity. Deficiency syndromes tend to be associated with chronic illness and may involve Deficient *yin*, *yang*, *qi*, or Blood. Excess syndromes tend to be associated with invading pathogens or some sort of organ problem leading to excess Phlegm, Dampness, or Blood Stagnation.

Cold syndromes involve cold limbs, aching joints, with watery catarrh or diarrhea.

Finally the doctor identifies whether the problem is *yin* or *yang*: Interior, Cold and Deficiency syndromes are *yin* while Exterior, Heat and Excess ones are *yang*. Typically, *yin* syndromes involve weakened *yang*, pathogenic Cold, reduced energy metabolism and insufficient Heat; disorders of Blood or the *zang* organs are also *yin*. *Yang* syndromes involve dominant internal Heat, *yang qi*, or increased energy metabolism; disorders involving *qi* of the *fu* organs are also *yang*.

REFINING THE DIAGNOSIS

Having applied the Eight Guiding Principles, the Chinese doctor can then further clarify the diagnosis depending on the initial identification.

For internal diseases, for example, the state of both *qi* and Blood need to be considered as there could be Deficiency or Stagnation, adverse flow of *qi*, or "toxic Heat" in the Blood.

Next any problems with the *zang-fu* organs involved need to be accurately identified; again these are classified as Excess or Deficiency problems. Some heart diseases or anemia, for example, would be classified as due to Deficiency of Heart *yin* or Heart Blood, while chronic bronchitis might be associated with an Excess syndrome caused by Wind-Cold invading the Lung.

The doctor may also apply the Theory of the six Channels: problems associated with *taiyin*, *shaoyin*, and *jueyin* are described as syndromes of the *yin* Channels, while those involving *yangming*, *taiyang*, and *shaoyang* are *yang*. The Channels are associated with either Interior, Exterior or both Interior and Exterior disorders, so by considering a patient's symptoms the doctor can identify the affected Channel, which then helps pinpoint the organs affected as well as whether the problem is Interior or Exterior. It also helps to predict the likely progression of the illness as the Channels are linked so the doctor can understand which organ may next be affected as the illness progresses.

Other diagnostic techniques focus on specific groups of diseases. The "Theory of *wei*, *qi*, *ying*, and *xue*," for example, was developed by Ye Tianshi (1667—1746) in his book *Wen Re Lun (On Febrile Disease)*, and helps to identify syndromes associated with pathogenic Heat. A *wei* syndrome involves a superficial attack on the body's surface, *qi* further involves the body's defence mechanisms, *ying* is an attack on the body's system of processing and distributing nutrients, while *xue* is Heat attacking the Blood. These four stages define the progression of attack by pathogenic Heat (infectious disease).

Differentiating Damp-Heat syndromes in infectious diseases uses the "Theory of the Triple Burner" developed by Wu Jutong (1758—1836) in the *Wen Bing Tiao Bian (Treatise on Differentiation and Treatment of Seasonal Warm*

Diseases) completed in 1798. This argues that epidemic diseases are either Warm-Heat or Damp-Heat. Damp-Heat diseases, largely confined to the *wei* and *qi* stages, which penetrate the *san jiao* (Triple Burner). From the patient's symptoms it is possible to identify which part of the *san jiao*—lower, middle, or upper—is affected and so deliver the appropriate treatment.

With both these theories it is worth remembering that doctors of the 17th and 18th centuries were much preoccupied with epidemic and infectious disorders, such as plague, smallpox, typhoid, or cholera that could often be fatal. Today, these "febrile diseases" are more likely to be treated with antibiotics.

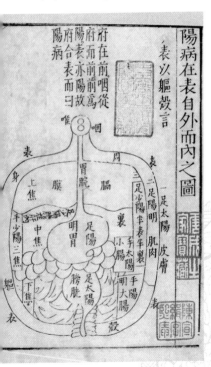

The Chinese view of digestion is very different to modern understanding, involving the Spleen and *san jiao*.

IDENTIFYING DISHARMONIES

The aim of the various diagnostic techniques is to use the Eight Guiding Principles in order to identify how the *zang-fu* organs are affected by external or internal pathogens and thus what the appropriate treatment may be.

External diseases are superficial and most commonly involve Wind, Damp, and Cold affecting the Lung, producing symptoms that Westerners describe as a common cold but in Chinese terms would be classified as Wind and/or Cold and/or Damp invading the Lung. A severe common cold may see Wind, Cold, or Damp moving into the Lungs causing symptoms that Westerners might call "flu-like."

The other *zang* organs are more likely to be affected by internal causes such as the seven emotions,

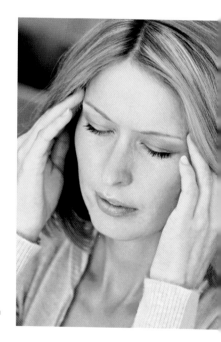

Headaches may have a variety of causes in Chinese medicine.

or by a failure to treat external pathogens in the early stages.

Internal disorders commonly involve Heat, Damp, and Cold with Wind which may be blamed for causing blockages in the Channels leading to pain. Too much Heat in the Heart, for example, can upset Blood circulation and mental activities since these are controlled by the Heart. Emotional disorders can be caused as well since the Heart stores Spirit, so disharmony can lead to insomnia and confusion.

Too much Heat in the Liver can lead to a Flaring of Liver Fire with excessive anger and irritability; it could damage Liver *yin* or interfere with the regular flow of *qi* since this is another Liver function. The Blood can be affected, since the Liver stores Blood.

Too much Damp in the Spleen can interfere with its ability to transport and transform fluids leading to digestive disorders and problems with urinary functions. Spleen Deficiency can cause a build-up of

Phlegm that can cause problems elsewhere in the system.

The Kidney can typically be affected by an excess of Cold and Damp, which can lead to Kidney *yang* Deficiency, while too much Heat can damage Kidney *yin*. If Kidney *qi* is weakened then Lung disorders such as asthma can follow since the Kidney helps the Lung to manage respiration. Kidney Deficiency also upsets water regulation leading to diarrhea or pain in the bones.

In theory, these imbalances will be identified by the physician during the examination, and appropriate treatment—including herbal brews, acupuncture, exercise routines, or dietary advice—can then be given. Treatment is designed to strengthen the body and restore balance, and regular monitoring is needed to see how the patient reacts to the changing stages of the disorder as recovery progresses.

CHINESE SYNDROMES

While it is fairly easy for non-experts to understand such concepts as *qi* Deficiency, there are many syndrome names that seem confusing and incomprehensible. They date back to a time when fatal epidemic diseases were far more prevalent than they are today. Illnesses that are now successfully treated with modern drugs, or have been virtually eradicated thanks to vaccination programs, were of largely unknown cause and often fatal in earlier centuries.

Many of the names developed as descriptions of illnesses and still appear in Chinese herbals or may be found on websites selling Chinese patent remedies. Some of the syndromes that are commonly mentioned include:

Abandoned Syndrome (*tuo zheng*) is typified by heavy sweating, sagging jaw, closed eyes, incontinence, and a small thin pulse. This is due to severe injury to *qi*, Blood, *yin*, and *yang* so that the patient is "abandoned" by their essential *qi*. It is likely to be caused by a stroke (cerebrovascular accident).

"Cock–crow diarrhea" (*wu geng xie*) has symptoms of abdominal pain and wind early in the morning, relieved by evacuation of the bowels and is associated with Deficient Kidney *yang*.

Fire Poison (*huo du*) is any disorder with severe Heat and Poison where the patient feels sick; usually caused by boils, abscesses, carbuncles, or soft tissue inflammations.

Indeterminate Gnawing Hunger (*cao za*) is an unpleasant sensation of apparent pain and hunger when there is neither and is associated with peptic ulcers and gastritis.

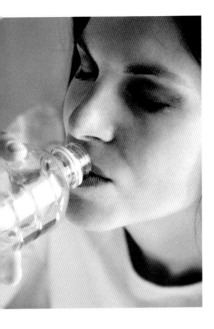

Extreme thirst, a common symptom of diabetes—classified by the ancients as "Wasting and Thirsting Syndrome."

restlessness that may be due to frustration caused by Constrained Liver *qi* or excessive worrying caused by Deficient Spleen. In the West it would have been described as "hysteria."

Steaming Bone Syndrome (*gu zheng*) is a deficient *yin* fever characterized by a sensation of heat radiating from the bones to the skin, with night sweats, breathing problems, and disturbed sleep; often associated with pulmonary tuberculosis.

Wasting and Thirsting Syndrome (*xiao ke bing*) is typified by extreme and constant thirst, emaciation, and excessive urination and now equated with diabetes.

Painful Obstruction (*bi*) are disorders associated with blockages in the Channels (meridians) usually associated with external pathogens. *Bi* syndrome is most commonly associated with arthritis but may also affect any of the *zang-fu* organs.

Restless Organ Syndrome (*zang zao*) is typified by inappropriate behavior, insomnia, mania, and

APPLYING CHINESE DIAGNOSIS

Common ailments defined in Western terms can take on a whole new meaning when Chinese medicine diagnostics are applied.

COMMON COLD

Common colds with catarrh, sneezing, headache, chills, cough, or sore throat are usually treated in the West with an assortment of products providing symptomatic relief—Aspirin, cough mixtures, nasal sprays, and so on.

In Chinese theory such colds are regarded as caused by external pathogens becoming more severe or flu-like if the pathogens are strong enough to invade the Channels. The nature of the pathogen determines the symptoms the sufferer will endure and these will guide the doctor in prescribing the correct remedy to support the body's anti-pathogenic *qi*.

The cold's onset is often linked to abnormal weather so the doctor notes climatic conditions when the cold began. Obviously, modern Chinese medicine practitioners accept that contagious infections can cause colds not just external "evils," but treatment is still based on an analysis of symptoms and the body's reaction to the pathogen rather than taking a single one-size-fits-all approach.

TREATMENTS

Colds due to pathogenic Wind-Cold, for example, generally involve chills, watery catarrh, an absence of sweating, sneezing, headaches, aching joints, ticklish throat, cough with little sputum, a pale coating to the tongue, and a floating or tight

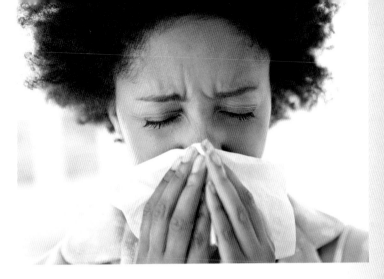

pulse. Such colds are treated with warming, pungent herbs such as *gui zhi* (cinnamon twigs) or *zi su zi* (perilla seeds).

A cold due to Wind-Heat would be typified by a high fever, sweating, headache, thick nasal catarrh, a dry and sore throat, cough with sticky sputum, a yellow tongue coating with the tongue red at the edges and tip, and a floating, rapid pulse. Appropriate herbs this time are pungent and cool such as *bo he* (field mint), *niu bang zi* (burdock seeds) or *ju hua* (chrysanthemum flowers).

In Chinese theory common colds have many different causes.

Seasonal colds have their distinct symptoms and remedies. A cold due to pathogenic Dryness in autumn, for example, is characterized by fever, chills, headache, a dry unproductive cough, thirst, dry mouth and nose, minimal saliva, red tongue with thin coating, and a floating and rapid pulse. Remedies may include herbs that are more moistening to clear the Dryness as well as soothe the Lung and increase saliva, such as *sang ye* (mulberry leaf) or *jie geng* (balloon flower root).

PREMENSTRUAL SYNDROME

For many women premenstrual syndrome (PMS) is a monthly nightmare with symptoms that can include bouts of anger, irritability, and depression, abdominal bloating, diarrhea and/or constipation, food cravings, breast swelling or tenderness, headaches, and insomnia. In Western medicine the symptoms are often blamed on hormonal imbalance.

In Chinese theory the Liver stores Blood and is thus closely associated with menstruation. It also regulates the flow of *qi* so any problems with the Liver are likely to impede *qi* flow leading to Obstructions and Stagnation elsewhere in the body.

During the examination a Chinese doctor will ask questions about the menstrual blood—if dark and clotted, for example, this could indicate

Abdominal bloating can be a symptom of premenstrual syndrome.

Stagnation of *qi* and Blood: *qi* moves Blood so if *qi* Stagnates so does Blood. Such Stagnation in the lower abdomen can be caused by some sort of damage to Liver *qi*. Breast swelling can also be traced back to

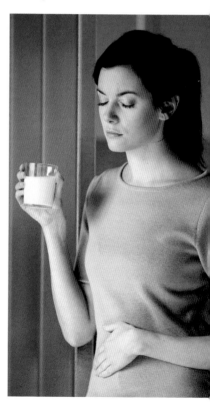

Liver problems with branch collaterals of the foot *jueyin* meridian (the Liver Channel) supplying the nipple while the Stomach meridian also crosses the breasts.

The Liver is also associated with the emotion anger and the sound of shouting. PMS is often followed by a painful period—another indication of Stagnating *qi* and Blood.

A SIGN OF CONGESTION

Rather than being hormonal, Chinese medicine regards PMS as a sign of Congested Liver *qi*. From the five-phase model the Chinese doctor will also know that an overforceful Liver can impede Spleen function, weakening the digestion and distribution of nutrients, which can affect the appetite and lead to food cravings, nausea, or fluid retention as the normal circulation systems fail. So as well as Liver *qi* Congestion the PMS sufferer may also have some form of Spleen Deficiency.

TREATMENTS

As well as herbal brews and acupuncture, treatment might include exercise since, in Chinese theory, too much sitting can lead to Congestion and Stagnation. The Spleen can also be weakened by too much cold food so the patient may be advised to eat warm foods and avoid cold drinks or excessive fluid intake since weakened Spleen can lead to Fluid Stagnation and Internal Damp problems.

Herbal treatment could include remedies to help normalize Liver *qi* and nourish Blood, such as *dang gui* (Chinese angelica), *bai shao yao* (white peony root), or *chai hu* (thorowax root).

ARTHRITIS

Western medicine regards arthritis as a joint inflammation generally treated with anti-inflammatory drugs. There are many types of arthritis including osteoarthritis, caused by wear-and-tear damage to the joints, and rheumatoid arthritis, an auto-immune disease where the body itself destroys the joint lining.

In Chinese theory, arthritis—referred to as *bi* syndrome—is seen as caused by pathogenic Wind, Cold, Dampness, or Heat leading to obstructions of the meridians and sluggish circulation of *qi* and Blood. Symptoms can include numbness and heaviness of the muscles, tendons or joints as well as joint swelling and restricted movement.

TYPES OF *BÌ* SYNDROME

There are various types of *bi* syndrome depending on the invading pathogens and why they have been so successful. Sufferers are likely to have low resistance (weakened *wèi qì*) that allows pathogens to enter: those with *yang* Deficiency would be more susceptible to Wind, Cold, and Damp; those with *yin* Deficiency or over-dominant *yang* would be more likely to suffer Wind-Heat-Damp *bi* syndrome. In the Wind-Damp-Heat variety joints are red, hot, and swollen. If Wind is dominant then the pains shift between joints, if Cold is the predominant pathogen then the pain is localized and severe, while Dampness increases the sensations of numbness and heaviness.

Initially the problem is seen as exterior and superficial, but if untreated the pathogens enter the interior and the severity increases. *Bi* syndrome that is fixed rather than producing migratory pains is more akin to the Western definition of rheumatoid arthritis, while the Wind-Cold-Damp variety is more comparable with osteoarthritis.

Arthritis, especially rheumatoid arthritis, can affect the joints of the fingers.

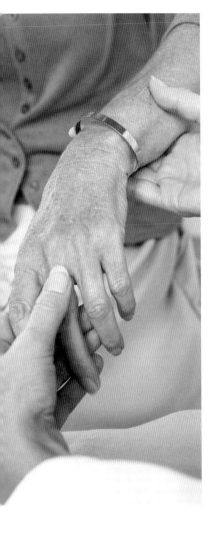

TREATMENTS

Treatment is focused on expelling the invading pathogens followed by strengthening the Blood and *zang-fu* organs, especially Spleen, Liver, and Kidney since these are the organs associated with, respectively, muscles, tendons, and bones. Treatment may also include herbs or acupuncture to encourage Blood circulation and dispel any stasis. Severe Damp can also give rise to Phlegm so, again, if this was present, additional remedies would be used.

Herbs used for the Cold types of arthritis include *ma huang* (ephedra), *gui zhi* (cinnamon twigs), *fang feng* (siler root), and various types of specially prepared aconite (*fu zi*), an extremely toxic plant little used in the West. Tonic remedies like *ren shen* (Korean ginseng) and *huang qi* (milk vetch) may also be added.

HIGH BLOOD PRESSURE

While in the West high blood pressure is generally treated with beta-blockers, vasodilators, diuretics, and a host of other pills and potions, Chinese theory focuses on correcting the imbalances that may be causing the condition.

Causes can be:

- emotional problems, with worry affecting the Spleen leading to stagnation of vital energy in the Liver, which in turn causes a Flaring of Liver Fire.

- improper diet with too much greasy food and alcohol causing imbalances in Spleen and Stomach, with failure to transport water and nutrients and a resulting increase in Phlegm.

- overwork or ageing with a reduction in Kidney essence that affects the Liver, again causing Flaring of Liver Fire

Other causes include problems with Phlegm blocking the Heart Channel or Heart Deficiency causing Stagnation of *qi* and Blood.

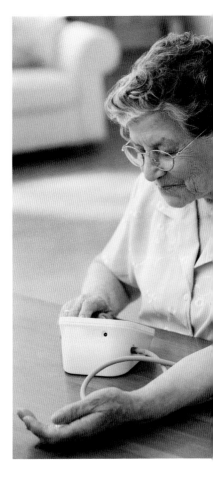

Monitoring their own blood pressure has become a preoccupation for many people in the West.

SYMPTOMS AND TREATMENT

The symptoms and treatment of each condition vary significantly. Flaring of Liver Fire, for example, may cause dizziness, headache, blurred vision, a red flushed face, a bitter taste in the mouth, irritability, numbness in lips and tongue, insomnia, with a red tip to the tongue, yellow coating, and taut and rapid pulse, as well as raised blood pressure. Treatment focuses on calming the Liver and clearing the endogenous Wind, which is fanning the Fire. Herbs that cool and sedate Liver Fire and clear Heat such as *long dan cao* (gentian), *huang qin* (baikal skullcap root) and *zhi zi* (gardenia fruits) might be included in remedies.

If poor diet has resulted in a build-up of Phlegm, then nausea and vomiting with an oppressive feeling in the stomach, lack of appetite, disturbed and dreamy sleep and a cough with mucous-like sputum might be symptoms. The tongue will still have a red tip but is otherwise pale with a slimy yellow coating and the pulse is taut and slippery. Treatment aims to subdue endogenous Wind but is also focused on clearing Phlegm with warm, drying herbs like *huang lian* (golden thread) and *huang qin* (baikal skullcap root).

If Deficient vital essence of Kidney and Liver is to blame then symptoms may include dizziness, tinnitus, headache, a flushed face on exertion, dry mouth, weight loss, weakness in the lower back and legs, a deep red tongue with little coating, and a thready, taut pulse. Here treatment is focused on replenishing vital essence with tonic herbs including *di huang* (Chinese foxglove), *shan zhu yu* (dogwood fruits), or *mu dan pi* (tree peony root bark).

DIARRHEA

While diarrhea is generally seen in the West as a symptom of food poisoning, irritable bowel syndrome, gastroenteritis, or some other disorder, in Chinese theory it can also have a number of other causes and appropriate remedies.

External pathogens are often to blame—Cold, Dampness, and Summer Heat are all seen as potential causes of Spleen dysfunction with a failure of the usual mechanisms for transporting and distributing water and nutrients. There could also be poor Spleen and Stomach function caused by improper diet; too much fatty, sweet,

"Cock-crow diarrhea" is typified by an early morning rush for the bathroom with abdominal pain that is soon relieved.

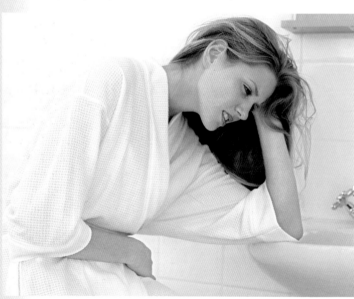

cold, raw, or infected food, or emotional strain could be a factor causing stagnation of Liver *qi* that damages the Spleen. In chronic illness, too, Kidney *qi* can be weakened, which in turn fails to strengthen the Spleen.

Diagnosis includes examining the precise pattern of the diarrhea and stools: loose, watery stools with indigestion suggests pathogenic Cold; stools that are dark and smell particularly unpleasant accompanied by a burning sensation in the anus suggest pathogenic Heat.

TREATMENTS

The aim of treatment is to clear the pathogen with supportive herbs: warm, drying remedies in the case of pathogenic Cold and cool, often bitter tasting herbs if Heat is to blame.

Diarrhea due to Spleen weakness generally involves undigested food in the stool due to a failure of the digestive system. Weak Spleen may also involve lack of appetite, lethargy, a feeling of oppression in the area around the stomach. The tongue will be pale with a white coating and the pulse weak and thready. Here treatment is aimed at reinforcing the Spleen's vital energy using tonic herbs such as *dang shen* (bellflower root) and remedies to clear Damp and normalize function like the fungus *fu ling* (tuckahoe).

If Kidney weakness is to blame, then the condition generally manifests as "cock-crow diarrhea" in the early morning with abdominal pains relieved when passing stools, and often cold limbs, lower back pain and weak knees. The tongue is pale with a white coating and the pulse deep and thready. Treatment aims to strengthen both Kidney and Spleen. A classic herbal remedy in this case is *si shen wan* ("pills of four miraculous drugs") that contains *bu gu zi* (scuffy pea seeds), *wu zhu yu* (evodia fruits), *rou dou kou* (nutmeg), and *wu wei zi* (schizandra fruits).

LOW BACK PAIN OR LUMBAGO

Backache is one of those common ailments that affects many people. In Western medicine a mechanical cause is generally sought—as wear-and-tear on vertebra, misaligned discs, sprained muscles, or trapped nerves; urinary tract, kidney, or fallopian tube inflammations may also be blamed.

SYMPTOMS AND TREATMENTS

In Chinese theory there are also several possible causes of low back pain. It could be caused by Damp-Cold entering the lumbar region and impairing the smooth flow of *qi* and Blood. Typically, there is increased pain on cold, wet days that is not relieved by bed rest, although the pain is relieved by warmth in the lumbar region. There is a slimy white coating to the tongue and deep slow pulse. Treatment is aimed at clearing the Cold and Damp and improving *qi* and Blood flow with herbs such as *fu ling* (tuckahoe), *bai zhu* (white atractylodes), and *du huo* (pubescent angelica).

Low back pain could also be related to Damp-Heat—both exogenous or endogenous—entering the Channels and causing obstructions. Symptoms include pain with a burning sensation and a bitter taste in the mouth. The tongue has a slimy yellow coating and the pulse is soft and rapid. Treatment is with cooling, dry herbs such as *huang bai* (cork tree bark) and *yi yi ren* (Job's tears seeds).

The pain may be related to weakened Kidney *jīng*, possibly associated with the normal run-down of essence in old age or excessive sexual activity. Pain may be relieved by pressure; symptoms could also include weakness in the legs and knees, dizziness, tinnitus, cold limbs, and a pale tongue with white coating and a deep, thready pulse. Tonic herbs for the Kidney in this case are *gou qi zi* (wolfberry fruits) and *shan zhu yu* (dogwood fruits).

Finally, low back pain may be related to *qi* and Blood Stagnation caused by traumatic injury or chronic illness. The

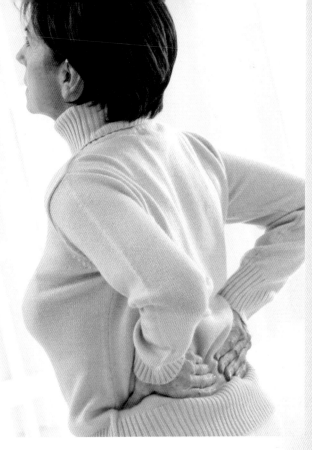

pain is likely to be sharp and stinging and is made worse by movement and pressure. The tongue will be dark red with a choppy pulse. Treatment is designed to normalize the Blood circulation and remove Blood Stagnation. Typical herbal remedies

Low back pain is a common complaint which Western medicine also sees as a mechanical problem.

will include *dang gui* (Chinese angelica), *chuan xiong* (Szechuan lovage), and *hong hua* (safflower).

CHINESE THERAPEUTICS

The various therapies used in Chinese medicine are believed to have originated in different parts of the country, with acupuncture coming from the South and East, herbs from the West, and heat treatments from the cold North.

Today, herbal remedies and acupuncture are perhaps the most familiar forms of Chinese medical treatment, while over the centuries Taoist philosophers and later interpreters have extended the therapeutic options. Some Chinese health therapists describe the total range of traditional medicine options as the "Eight Strands of Brocade" (*pa chin hsien*), which are generally given as:

- *chen tuan* diagnosis
- *ts'ao yao* herbal therapy
- *chang ming* diet therapy
- *hsia chen pien* acupuncture
- *wen chiech'u* thermology including moxibustion and use of poultices

- *tien chen* acupressure or spot pressing
- *tui na* or *anmo* massage
- *chili nung* the spiritual path; the use of meditation (*hsiang mo*) and *qi* control in healing

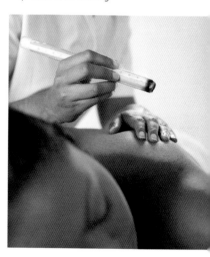

Moxibustion is one of the heat treatments included in the Eight Strands of Brocade.

Some exponents of the "Eight Pieces of Brocade" model replace diagnosis with *ti yu* physical exercise. Others speak of the "Eight Limbs" of treatment and health, which comprise: meditation; exercise; diet; bodywork or massage; herbalism; acupuncture; cosmology and astrology; and geomancy or *feng shui*.

The first six of these "eight limbs" are discussed in the following sections, while the last two—astrology and geomancy—are not always considered as aspects of Chinese medicine in the West although they can be relevant for some. *Feng shui* (literally "wind water") is well known outside China as a technique for designing houses and interior decorations to maximize good fortune, wealth, and health.

FENG SHUI

Although *feng shui* means "wind water," it is also about creating an environment where people can live in harmony with their surroundings or as one traditional definition puts it: "the art of adapting the residences of the living and the dead so as to co-operate and harmonize the local currents of the cosmic breath."

Like other forms of geomancy, *feng shui* is based on the theory that energy lines exist within the Earth—as the meridians do within the body—and these can be strengthened or damaged by the way mankind interacts with the landscape. The theory is popularly extended to suggest that hanging crystals and wind chimes in certain parts of the house or ensuring there is a bowl of fish at another will bring prosperity.

From a health perspective such practicalities, inherent in traditional *feng shui*, of ensuring that, for example, doors face away from prevailing winds and that homes are protected from excesses of Heat or Cold by good design have clear benefits.

CHINESE ASTROLOGY

In Tibetan medicine, which draws on both the Chinese and Ayurvedic traditions, astrology is an important aspect of diagnosis with the need for careful chart-making to compare the positions of the stars when the patient was born and when the illness began.

This approach is less common in traditional Chinese medicine as practiced today, although some therapists believe that the signs of the zodiac can influence health and tendencies for certain strengths and weaknesses.

Chinese astrology is based on a 12-year cycle of animals (*sheng xiào*): rat, ox, tiger, rabbit, dragon, snake, horse, goat, monkey, rooster, dog, and pig. The year itself is based on a lunar calendar so it varies in length. The year from February 15, 2010 to February 2, 2011 is a tiger year, from February 3, 2011 to January 22, 2012 a rabbit year, and so on.

ANIMALS AND ELEMENTS

This 12-year animal cycle is actually a 60-year sequence as the five "elements" of Chinese theory—wood, fire, earth, metal, and water—are

---

YIN/YANG AND ELEMENT ASPECTS

Matching the Chinese lunar year with the calendar year can be complex but as a general guide years ending in:

0 are *yang* metal

1 are *yin* metal

2 are *yang* water

3 are *yin* water

4 are *yang* wood

5 are *yin* wood

6 are *yang* fire

7 are *yin* fire

8 are *yang* earth

9 are *yin* earth

---

also applied in turn to each of the animals to give, for example, a "fire dragon" or "metal tiger" year, each with its own characteristics. The predominant element for each year links through the five-element model to suggest which of the *zang-fu* organs may dominate and thus where potential imbalances could lie.

In addition, some years are *yin* and others *yang* giving a predominant energy both to those born at that time and the ailments most likely to occur then.

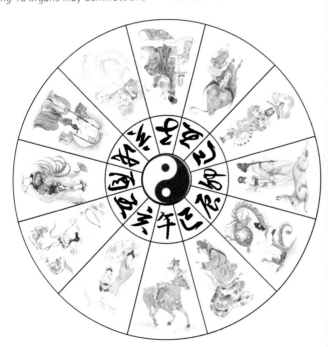

The animals linked to each year were once believed to influence health.

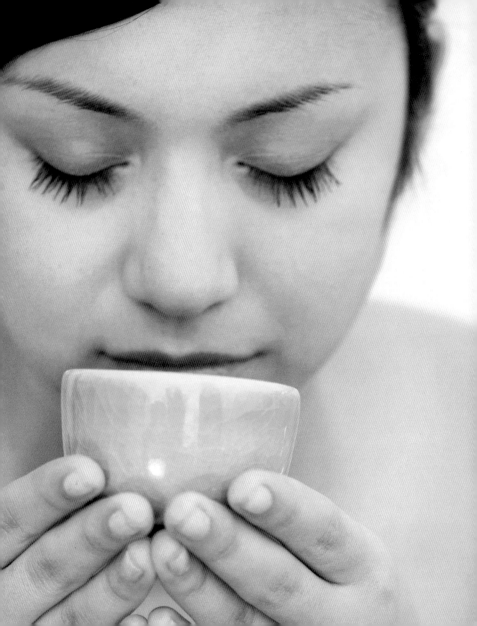

Part 3

CHINESE
MATERIA MEDICA

TYPES OF CHINESE HERBAL REMEDIES

Herbal remedies form the basis of traditional Chinese therapeutics: while acupuncture or massage are seen by many Westerners as more significant therapies, herbs will be prescribed in almost all cases and are regarded as the physician's most important tool. Herbs in Chinese theory can also include far more than plants: animal parts, minerals, fungi, human hair, insects, or even various animal droppings have all been used as medicine over the centuries.

The earliest herbal, the *Shen Nong Ben Cao Jing* (*The Divine Farmer's Herb Classic*) was written around CE 200, although it is believed to have existed in oral tradition for several thousand years before that. It lists 365 herbs including many that are still in use today. *Ma huang* (ephedra), for example, is still used to treat asthma and gave us the drug ephedrine, while the classic text refers to *dang gui* (Chinese angelica) as suitable for regulating menstruation: it is now sold as an over-the-counter remedy in Western shops for this very purpose.

HERBAL CATEGORIES

Over the centuries, Chinese scholars identified more healing remedies; the renowned Li Shi Zhen publishing his *Ben Cao Gan Mu* in the 1590s with its impressive listings of some 1,892 remedies made up into more than 11,000 different combinations. The remedies are grouped into such categories as woods, weeds, fruits, and so on, and listed by the Mandarin Chinese name for each "drug."

Modern Western *materia medica* are very precise in identifying the individual plants by standard botanical name but China is a large country and many of the plants growing in the sub-tropical south are very different from those growing in the cooler north. Different plants from the various regions may have similar therapeutic properties and be used in the same way, so it is possible for several unrelated botanical species to share the same Mandarin "drug" name.

This can seem very confusing to Westerners. Two quite different species of duckweed, for example, (*Spirodela polyrrhiza* and *Lemma minor*) are both called *fu ping* and used to treat common colds caused by Wind and Heat. Similarly, *fang ji*— a pungent remedy used to relieve the pain caused by Wind and Dampness in rheumatic and arthritic disorders—can be derived from *Stephania*, *Aristolochia*, or *Cocculus* species. *Aristolochia* species are highly toxic and can be fatal if misused so in restricting the use of *fang ji*, Western regulators also deny access to other safer remedies.

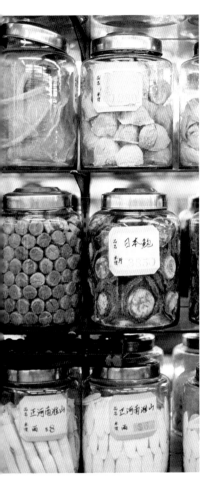

The Chinese "herbal" repertoire also includes shells, insects, minerals, and animal parts.

DIFFERENT NAMES FOR DIFFERENT PARTS

Equally confusing for non-Mandarin speakers is that different parts of the same plant can also have quite different Chinese names: cinnamon, for example, can be either *gui zhi* (twigs) or *rou gui* (bark); rather simpler is the white mulberry tree (*Morus alba*), which gives rise to *sang bai pi* (bark), *sang zhi* (twigs), *sang shen* (fruit), and *sang ye* (leaves), *sang pia xiao* is the steamed and dried egg case of the praying mantis laid on mulberry leaves, used to replenish Kidney *yang*, while *sang ji sheng* is mulberry mistletoe.

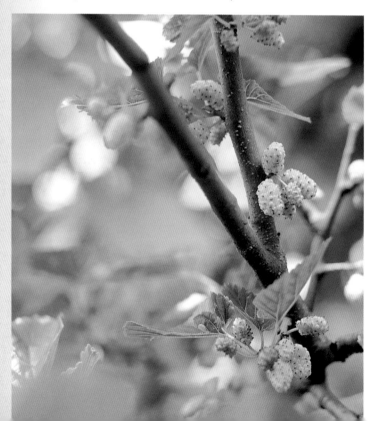

DIFFERENT PROCESSES

Plants can also be processed in different ways giving rise to further naming combinations: *di huang* is the root of the Chinese foxglove but *sheng di huang* is the fresh or dried root while *shu di huang* is a cooked or "prepared" version.

DIFFERENT COMBINATIONS

While Western herbalists tend to mix different plant extracts together on an ad hoc basis to treat each individual patient, Chinese medicine details many thousands of standard formulae—11,000 in Li Shi Zhen's 16th-century text—that are used as the basis of prescribing. Traditional Chinese medicine practitioners know hundreds of these combinations by heart and may use the basic combination, or amend it very slightly for their patients. The same

All parts of the white mulberry tree are used in Chinese medicine.

formulations are also sold as ready-made products, some of which are available as over-the-counter remedies in the West and are regularly used by Western-trained acupuncturists to augment treatments.

The various herbs in each prescription play quite different roles. These include:

- the emperor or chief—the principal therapeutic herbs
- the minister or deputy—herbs that support and strengthen the key plants
- a messenger or assistant—based on the directional properties of the plants to "target" the prescription to particular meridians or parts of the body
- ambassadors, helpers or harmonizers—auxiliary and/or correcting herbs that counter any toxic effects of the major ingredients or deal with secondary symptoms in the condition

ANIMAL PARTS

While a modern Western herbal is invariably a list of plants, Chinese herbal medicine still includes an assortment of animal parts, shells, and minerals used in treatments since the days of Shen Nong.

Western practitioners of traditional Chinese medicine try to avoid using many of these products since some are from endangered species or involve cruelty to animals. Others, in modern scientific terms, are poorly researched and are thus used with caution, if at all. The same does not apply to Chinese-made over-the-counter herbal products that can be bought on the Internet. These will often include animal parts listed either by their Chinese or zoological names, which often mean very little to the non-expert.

ANIMAL PARTS COMMONLY FOUND IN CHINESE REMEDIES

Xiong dan (Ursus arctos) is bear's gall bladder, used to clear Heat and Fire Poisons, and included in remedies for hepatitis associated with Liver Fire.

Hu gu (Panthera tigris) is tiger bone, used to disperse Wind-Cold and strengthen the sinews and bones. It

Rare species are still sometimes used in Chinese medicine.

is included in remedies for joint pain and stiffness associated with Wind Dampness.

Ye ming sha (Vespertillos murinus) is bat feces, used to clear Heat in the Liver associated with night blindness.

Xi jiao (Rhinoceros bicornis **or** *R. unicornis)* is rhinoceros horn, used to clear Heat, and Fire Poisons and cool Blood.

Hou zao (Macaca mulatta) are macaque gall stones, used to clear Phlegm, Heat, and Fire Poisons.

Ju nei jin (Gallus gallus domesticus) is chicken gizzard lining, used for food stagnation.

E jiao (Equus asinus) is gelatine made from donkey hide. This is used to nourish the Blood, stop bleeding, soothe the Lung, and nourish *yin.*

Chuan shan jia (Manis pentadactyla) are pangolin scales, used to disperse Congealed Blood, expel Wind Dampness and reduce swelling; used for painful joints and abdominal swellings.

Lu rong (Cervis nippon) is velvet from young deer antlers. It is used to tonify Kidney *yang, qi,* and Blood; included in many tonic formulae.

Ge jie (Gekko gecko) is gecko, used to tonify Kidney and Lung *yang;* included in various remedies for Kidney Deficient problems.

Hai gou shen (Callorhinus ursinus) are genitals of the male seal, used to strengthen *yang* and *jīng* and used for Deficient Kidney *yang* causing impotence.

hai ma (Hippocampus kelloggi) is seahorse, used to tonify the Kidneys and invigorate Blood; used for debility in the elderly.

di long (Pheretima aspergillum) is earthworm, used to clear Heat and Wind and to stop spasms and tremors; used for strokes, seizures, and traumatic injuries.

HERBAL REMEDIES

The properties of herbs used in traditional Chinese medicine reflect the various theories of five elements, *yin-yang*, and meridians.

Plants are defined in terms of property and taste. Herbs are also described as entering the meridians and have a direction inside the body with *yang* herbs tending to move upward and *yin* downward. Each attribute signifies further actions. Bitter herbs, for example, will reverse the upward flow of *qi* while hot

herbs dispel pathogenic Cold and strengthen *yang*. Traditional Chinese herbals tended to group plants either by type of remedy or by therapeutic action. Since Chinese names mean very little to Western readers, the listings in this section adopt this approach and group herbs by main action.

PROPERTIES OF HERBS AND ASSOCIATED SYNDROMES

Property	Action	Used for
Cold (*hán*)/ cool (*liang*)	To clear Heat To purge Fire To remove Toxins	Heat syndromes *Yang* syndromes Heat-toxin syndromes
Warm (*wen*)/hot (*rè*)	To warm the Interior To dispel Cold evils To strenghthen *yang*	Cold syndromes *Yin* syndromes *Yang* Deficiency syndromes
Neutral (*ping*)	Milder actions may both clear Heat and warm the Interior	All syndromes

TASTES OF HERBS AND ASSOCIATED SYNDROMES

Taste	Action	Used for
Pungent (*la*)	Dispersing/mobilizing	Superficial syndrome Wind syndrome Stagnant *qi* syndrome Stagnant Blood syndrome
Sour (*suān*), astringent	Contracting	Sweating associated with Deficiency Hemorrhage due to Deficiency Chronic diarrhea Involuntary urination
Sweet (*gan*)	Tonifying	Yin, yang or *qi* Deficient syndromes
	Clearing toxins	–
	Alleviating	Spasmodic pain
	Harmonizing the action of drugs	–
Salty (*xián*)	Softening/eliminating	Combating swellings (in lymphatic system) and other masses
	Lubricating the large intestine	Constipation
Bitter (*kū*)	Reversing upward motion of *qi*	Coughs, vomiting, constipation due to stagnation, problems with urination
	Drying Damp evil,	Water-Damp syndromes
	Activating *qi* and Blood motion	Coughs due to stagnant Lung *qi*, Stagnant Blood syndromes
Bland	Diuresis	Water-Damp syndromes

TAKING HERBAL REMEDIES

Traditionally, most Chinese herbal remedies are made into decoctions known as *tāng* (soup). Patients are given small paper bags containing each day's dosage; this is soaked with three cups of water (about 500 ml) for about 20–30 minutes, then simmered gently until the volume has reduced by about half (another 25–30 minutes). This mixture is then strained and the liquid is taken as a single dose on an empty stomach.

The quantities of herbs used each day are higher than in Western herbal medicine and, as a result, Chinese decoctions are usually a thick, dark brown with a strong, generally unpleasant taste that many Westerners find difficult to take. As well as decoctions, Chinese herbal formulae can also be powdered (*sàn*) or made into pills (*wán*). Pills, usually resembling small black ball bearings, are traditionally made by rolling powdered herbs with honey, and dosages are generally around six or eight pills at a time. Powders are generally stirred into water or wine. Some prescriptions are specifically

designed to be taken in pill form—such as *liù wèi dì huáng wán* (pills of six ingredients with Chinese foxglove) taken for Liver and Kidney *yin* Deficiency.

Herbal wines (*jiu*) are also used as tonic remedies with roots simply steeped in wine for several weeks and then taken in small doses on a daily basis.

ADAPTING TO WESTERN LIFESTYLES

Brewing the daily *tāng* is a time-consuming business for Western households; consequently, Western-

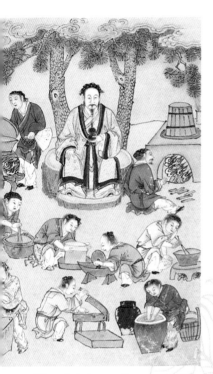

Chinese herbal preparations—soups, pills, and powders—have been made in much the same way for generations.

formulae in capsules, tablets, or as liquid extracts. These are easy, convenient and pleasant to take, although some purists would argue that they are not as effective as the traditional remedies.

A market has also developed for over-the-counter Chinese herbs used in non-traditional ways. Individual herbs are often available in tincture or fluid extract form in health food shops, while various blends of herbal powders or liquid extracts are sold under a variety of names designed to appeal to Western shoppers.

Traditional Chinese medicine very rarely uses a single herb as a remedy; the emphasis is always on tried-and-trusted formulae that have evolved over the centuries so taking a single herb is unusual. Equally, while many herbs are added to standard formulae to adapt the mix to a particular condition or syndrome, these are also well-defined and standardized combinations with little of the *ad hoc* approach to herbal remedies that are common in the West.

trained acupuncturists and many practitioners working in the West use alternative extracts.

Commercial producers now supply many of the traditional *tāng*

HERBS FOR EXTERIOR CONDITIONS

Exterior or superficial diseases (see pages 54–65) are caused by external "evils" such as Cold, Damp, or Wind-Heat. Typical symptoms include coughs, chills, fevers, or general muscle aches regarded in the West as typical of the "common cold." The herbs used to treat these conditions are described as "releasing the exterior." Herbs for Exterior conditions fall into two main groups—warm, pungent herbs for treating Cold conditions, and cold pungent herbs for treating Heat problems.

WARM PUNGENT HERBS

Warm pungent herbs are used where the chills are severe, fever is mild, and additional symptoms include headache, body and neck pains, and lack of thirst.

ACTIONS Antibacterial, antifungal, antiviral, analgesic, carminative, cardiotonic, diuretic.

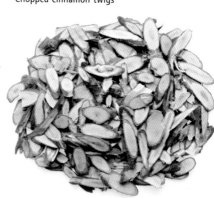

Chopped cinnamon twigs

Gui zhi cinnamon twigs

BOTANICAL NAME *Cinnamomum cassia*
TASTE Pungent, sweet
CHARACTER Warm
MERIDIANS Heart, Lung, Urinary Bladder

The twigs of Chinese cinnamon are a popular remedy for treating external Cold and Wind-Cold conditions. It is said to "warm the channels" and is included in prescriptions for some gynecological problems such as period pain associated with internal Cold. As a warming herb it is naturally *yang* and is used to improve the circulation of *yang qi* and strengthen Heart *yang*.

● *Gui zhi* should be avoided in feverish conditions, excess Heat or Fire, and in pregnancy.

● **HOW TO USE** For Exterior Cold it can be taken in teas and is often combined with *bai shao yao* (white peony), *sheng jiang* (fresh ginger), and *gan cao* (baked liquorice).

Zi su ye perilla leaf

BOTANICAL NAME *Perilla frutescens*
TASTE Pungent
CHARACTER Warm
MERIDIANS Lung, Spleen
ACTIONS Antibacterial, antitussive (anticoughing), diaphoretic (antiperspiring), expectorant

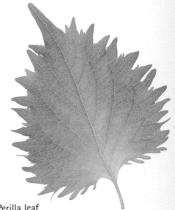
Perilla leaf

Perilla is familiar in the West as an ingredient in Chinese and Japanese cookery. The leaves are used to disperse Exterior Cold, especially Wind-Cold with coughs, and also to circulate Stomach and Spleen *qi* associated with *san jiao* disharmony. Perilla seeds are mainly used as a cough remedy to clear Phlegm.

● *Zi su ye* should be avoided for feverish diseases and *qi* Deficiency.

● **HOW TO USE** For Wind-Cold it can be taken in teas with *jie geng* (balloon flower) and is also made into a powder as *xiang su san*, which contains *chen pi* (tangerine peel), *xiang fu* (cyperus), and *gan cao* (baked liquorice).

Sheng jiang fresh ginger root

BOTANICAL NAME *Zingiber officinale*
TASTE Pungent
CHARACTER Warm
MERIDIANS Lung, Spleen, Stomach
ACTIONS Antiemetic, antispasmodic, antiseptic, carminative, circulatory stimulant, diaphoretic, expectorant, peripheral vasodilator, topically: rubefacient

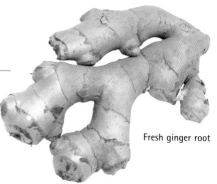

Fresh ginger root

Widely used both as a remedy in its own right and cooked with other herbs to reduce their toxicity, *sheng jiang* (fresh ginger) is used as a warming remedy for Wind-Cold. It is said to strengthen the *wei qi* and "release the Exterior." It also warms the middle *jiao* and is used for vomiting associated with Cold in the Stomach. Dried ginger (*gan jiang*) is a more warming remedy while the peel of fresh ginger root (*sheng jiang pi*) is used as a diuretic.

● Avoid ginger in Internal Heat syndromes.

● **HOW TO USE** For Wind-Cold *sheng jiang* is generally decocted with a little brown sugar added.

OTHER WARM PUNGENT HERBS

● *Ma huang* (*Ephedra sinensis*): ephedra stem is restricted in Europe.

● *Qing huo* (*Notopterygium incisium*): notopterygii root is commonly used when the condition also involves Dampness.

● *Fang feng* (*Ledebouriella sesloides*): siler root is mainly used for Wind-Cold and Wind-Damp linked to rheumatic disorders.

● *Bai zhi* (*Angelica dahurica*): dahurian angelica is mainly used to expel Wind.

● *Xi xin* (*Asarum siebaldi*): wild ginger is used to warm the Lungs and expel Cold and Wind.

● *Jing jie* (*Schizonepeta tenuifolia*): schizonepeta leaf and flower are mainly used for dispersing pathogenic Wind in Wind-Heat and Wind-Cold syndromes.

● *Xin yi hua* (*Magnolia liliflora*): magnolia flower is used to expel Wind and open the nasal passages.

COOL PUNGENT HERBS

These are used for Wind-Heat superficial syndromes where symptoms include relatively severe fevers with chills, dry, or sore throat, and thirst. Some can also be used for eye problems associated with Wind-Heat.

Bo he field mint

BOTANICAL NAME *Mentha arvensis*
TASTE Pungent
CHARACTER Cool
MERIDIANS Liver, Lung
ACTIONS Antibacterial, anti-inflammatory, antispasmodic, analgesic, diaphoretic

A key remedy for Wind-Heat problems especially where symptoms include headache and sore throat or eye problems, field mint is said to "let out" skin eruptions so is used for measles and other rashes. It helps to disperse Stagnant Liver *qi*.

● *Bo he* should be avoided in *yin* Deficiency and Excess Liver *qi*.

● **HOW TO USE** For Wind-Heat use with *niu bang zi* (burdock seeds) or combine in a powder with *lian qiao* (forsythia fruits) and *jin yin hua* (honeysuckle flowers). For Stagnant Liver *qi* a small amount is often included in formulae containing herbs like *bai shao yao* (white peony) and *chai hu* (thorowax root).

Field mint

Ju hua chrysanthemum flowers

BOTANICAL NAME *Dendranthema x grandiflorum*
TASTE Pungent, sweet, bitter
CHARACTER Cool
MERIDIANS Lung, Liver
ACTIONS Antibacterial, antifungal, antiviral, anti-inflammatory, hypotensive, peripheral vasodilator

One of China's most popular over-the-counter herbal teas, these are generally steamed before being dried, which removes much of the bitterness. *Ju hua* is used to clear pathogenic Wind-Heat and also used to clear Liver Heat. Since the Liver is associated with the eyes *ju hua* eases sore red eyes caused either by Wind-Heat in the Liver Channel or Liver Fire.

- *Ju hua* should be avoided in diarrhea and *qi* Deficiency
- **HOW TO USE** *Ju hua* is often used with *sang ye* (mulberry leaf) for pathogenic Heat affecting the upper *jiao* and with *shu di huang* (Chinese foxglove), *gou qi zi* (wolfberry fruits) or *bao shao yao* (white peony) for eye problems.

Chai hu thorowax root

BOTANICAL NAME *Bupleurum chinense*
TASTE Bitter, pungent
CHARACTER Slightly cold
MERIDIANS Liver, Gall bladder, Pericardium, *san jiao*
ACTIONS Antibacterial, antiviral, antimalarial, analgesic, anti-inflammatory, cholagogue, mild hypotensive, sedative

One of the herbs commonly used in China to treat malaria, it is regarded as a remedy for pathogenic

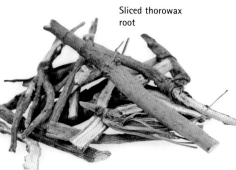

Sliced thorowax root

Wind-Heat, and an important treatment for dispersing stagnant Liver *qi* associated with gynecological disorders.

● *Chai hu* should be avoided in Liver Fire or *yin* Deficiency.

● **HOW TO USE** To disperse external evils that have entered the *shaoyang* Channel and becoming a more serious Internal problem. It is often combined with *huang qin* (baikal skullcap root), *ban xia* (pinellia), and *gan cao* (liquorice). For stagnant Liver qi it is commonly used with *bai shao yao* (white peony), *dang gui* (Chinese angelica), and *fu ling* (tuckahoe).

OTHER COLD PUNGENT HERBS

● *Niu bang zi* (*Arctium lappa*): burdock seed is mainly used for dispersing Wind-Heat and associated skin eruptions.

● *Sang ye* (*Morus alba*): mulberry leaf is used to expel Wind and clear Heat from the Lungs; also used for Heat or Wind in the Liver Channel causing eye problems.

● *Ge gen* (*Pueraria lobata*): kudzu vine root,is used to disperse pathogenic Wind-Heat and Wind-Cold and also to increase Spleen and Stomach *qi* where symptoms can include diarrhea.

● *Fu ping* (*Spirodela polyrrhiza* or *Lemna minor*): duckweed is one of the few cold and pungent herbs that is also diaphoretic; used for common colds, Wind rash, and measles.

HERBS TO CLEAR HEAT

Heat can be an External and Internal problem. Typical Heat symptoms include dry throat, red face or eyes, dark and scanty urine, dry stools, a rapid pulse, and yellow coating to the tongue. External Heat problems may include fever and chills, while Internal Heat is more likely to cause thirst, irritability, and feeling hot but without a chill or cold. Herbs to clear Internal Heat are all cold and often have a bitter taste. They are divided into five groups of herbs to: quell Fire; cool Blood; clear Heat and dry Dampness; clear Heat and Poisons; clear Summer Heat.

HERBS TO QUELL FIRE

These are some of the coldest herbs in the repertoire and are used for treating high fevers and heat in the Liver, Lungs, and Stomach. In Western terms they are known to be antimicrobial, anti-inflammatory, and antipyretic.

Shi gao gypsum

CHEMICAL NAME *Calcium sulphate* (often naturally occurring with iron or magnesium salts)
TASTE Sweet, pungent
CHARACTER Cold
MERIDIANS Lung, Stomach
ACTIONS Antipyretic, sedative, decreases the permeability of blood vessels, inhibits sweating, increases blood calcium levels

Gypsum is added to an herbal mixture as small broken pieces of rock. *Shi gao* is also used to clear excess Heat from the Lungs, characterized by coughing and wheezing; and also controls Stomach Fire that can cause toothache, painful gums, or headache.

● *Shi gao* should not be used in Deficient *yang* syndromes, where the Stomach is weak or if there are no signs of Heat or Dampness.

● **HOW TO USE** With other cold herbs in severe epidemic diseases where Heat has entered the interior affecting *qi* and Blood; with *shu di huang* (prepared Chinese foxglove) for headaches and toothaches caused by Internal Fire.

It is widely used to reduce Heat and quell Fire as well as to nurture yin and moisten Dry conditions.

● Avoid *zhi mu* if there is diarrhea.

● **HOW TO USE** *Zhi mu* is for conditions involving Heat and *yin* Deficiency. It is used in *er mu san* (fritillary and anemarrhena powder) for menopausal problems or in *gui zhi shao yao zhi mu tang* (decoction of cinnamon twig, peony, and anemarrhena) for certain types of arthritis. It is used with *xuan shen* (Ningpo figwort) and *sheng di huang* (Chinese foxglove) for mouth ulcers.

Zhi mu anemarrhena root

BOTANICAL NAME *Anemarrhena asphodeloides*

TASTE Bitter

CHARACTER Cold

MERIDIANS Lung, Stomach, Kidney

ACTIONS Antibacterial, diuretic, hypoglycemic, expectorant, antifungal, antipyretic

Sliced anemarrhena root

OTHER HERBS TO QUELL FIRE

● *Xia ku cao* (*Prunella vulgaris*) self-heal flower spike mainly used for treating Liver Fire.

● *Zhi zi* (*Gardenia jasminoides*) gardenia fruit used to drain Heat from the *san jiao* and cool Blood.

● *Lu gen* (*Phragmites communis*) reed rhizome used to clear Heat from the Lungs and Stomach and also generate Fluids.

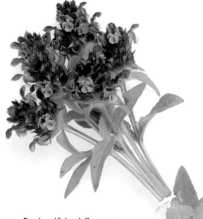

Fresh self-heal flowers

HERBS THAT COOL BLOOD

Symptoms associated with Heat in the Blood include rashes, spitting or vomiting blood, nosebleeds, and blood in the urine or stool.

Sheng di huang Chinese foxglove root (fresh or dried*)*

BOTANICAL NAME *Rehmannia glutinosa*
TASTE Sweet, bitter
CHARACTER Cold
MERIDIANS Heart, Liver, Kidney

ACTIONS Antibacterial, antifungal, diuretic, hypertensive, increases coagulation.

Chinese foxglove is used as either fresh or dried root (*sheng di huang*) and a cooked form made by stir-frying the sliced tubers in wine (*shu di huang*). *Sheng di huang* is used to clear Heat, cool the Blood, nourish *yin* and generate body fluids. It also "cools the upward flaring of Heart Fire" that can cause mouth and tongue sores and lead to insomnia and irritability. *Shu di huang* is an important Blood tonic.

● Both forms of *di huang* should be avoided if there is diarrhea; *sheng di huang* should not be taken if there is Deficient *yang* or Spleen and is best avoided in pregnancy.

● HOW TO USE *Sheng di huang* is combined with other cold herbs, such as *xuan shen* (Ningpo figwort) or *mu dan pi* (tree peony root bark) for treating feverish diseases that may be affecting Blood. With herbs such as *qing hao* (sweet wormwood) and *mu dan pi* it is used for *yin* Deficiency in the later stages of fevers.

Young Chinese foxglove plant

Xuan shen Ningpo figwort root

BOTANICAL NAME *Scrophularia ningpoensis*
TASTE Bitter, salty
CHARACTER Cold
MERIDIANS Lung, Stomach, Kidney
ACTIONS Antibacterial, antiviral, cardiotonic, hypotensive, hypoglycemic

Used for clearing pathogenic Heat that has entered the Blood and to nourish *yin*, it is particularly effective for dispelling nodules and detoxifying Fire Poisons.

● *Xuan shen* should be avoided with diarrhea.

● **HOW TO USE** *Xuan shen* combines well with *lian qiao* (forsythia fruits) for deep-seated abscesses and with *niu bang zi* (burdock seeds) for acute swellings in the throat. For irritant rashes it works well with *mu dan pi* (tree peony root bark).

OTHER HERBS TO COOL BLOOD

● *Mu dan pi* (*Paeonia suffruticosa*): tree peony root bark helps to invigorate Blood to clear Stagnation and congealed masses, and helps to clear ascending Liver fire.

● *Di gu pi* (*Lycium chinense*): wolfberry root bark is used to clear Deficient *yin* Fire and Heat.

HERBS TO CLEAR HEAT AND DRY DAMPNESS

Mainly used for Damp-Heat syndromes with symptoms that include problems with urination, diarrhea, eczema, or jaundice, these herbs are mostly cold and bitter and in conventional medical terms would be described as anti-inflammatory and antipyretic.

Huang qin baikal skullcap root

BOTANICAL NAME *Scutellaria baicalensis*
TASTE Bitter
CHARACTER Cold
MERIDIANS Lung, Heart, Stomach, Gall Bladder, Large Intestine
ACTIONS Antibacterial, antispasmodic, diuretic, febrifuge, lowers blood cholesterol

Mainly used to clear Damp-Heat and quell Fire, especially in the upper *jiao*, it also is said to "calm the fetus and pacify the womb" in conditions where the fetus is over-active and kicking due to Heat.

● Avoid *huang qin* where there are no true Heat and Dampness symptoms.

● **HOW TO USE** *Huang qin* is generally used with other cooling herbs like *huang lian* (Chinese golden thread) and *xuan shen* (Ningpo figwort) for feverish conditions with dry throat, insomnia, diarrhea, boils, or acute infections. It is used with *xia ku cao* (self-heal spikes) for excess Liver Fire and with remedies like *mu dan pi* (tree peony root bark) or *sheng di huang* (Chinese foxglove) where there is Heat in the Blood.

Huang bai cork tree bark

BOTANICAL NAME *Phellodendron amurense*
TASTE Bitter
CHARACTER Cold
MERIDIANS Kidney, Urinary Bladder
ACTIONS Antibacterial, cholagogue, diuretic, hypoglycemic, hypotensive, antipyretic

Huang bai is particularly effective for Damp-Heat in the lower *jiao* and is also used to quell Kidney Fire

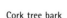

Cork tree bark

and drain Fire Poisons causing sores and skin lesions.

● *Huang bai* should be avoided if there is diarrhea or Stomach weakness.

● **HOW TO USE** *Huang bai* is combined with *shan yao* (Chinese yam) for urinary problems associated with Damp-Heat and with *chi shao yao* (red peony) where there is also Heat in the Blood. It is included in patent remedies including *er miao san* (powder of two effective ingredients) used to clear Heat and Dampness and *zhi bai di huang wan* (anemarrhena, cork tree, and pills of six herbs with Chinese foxglove) to replenish Kidney *yin*.

OTHER HERBS TO CLEAR HEAT AND DRY DAMPNESS

● *Huang lian* (*Coptis chinensis*): gold thread root is used for a wide range of Heat problems including dysentery, "marauding Hot Blood," excess Stomach Heat, mouth ulceration, boils, and abscesses.

● *Long dan cao* (*Gentiana scabra*): Chinese gentian root is used to drain Heat and Damp from the Liver and Gall Bladder Channels associated with red and swollen throat, eyes, and ears as well as to calm Liver Fire.

HERBS THAT CLEAR HEAT AND POISONS

Hot Poisons (*rè dú*) and Fire Poisons (*huǒ dú*) are typified by fevers, swellings, abscesses, and dysentery. These herbs are all cooling and most are known to be anti-inflammatory, antimicrobial or antiviral.

Jin yin hua honeysuckle flowers

BOTANICAL NAME *Lonicera japonica*
TASTE Sweet

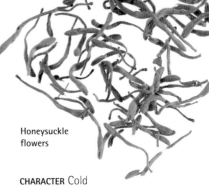

Honeysuckle flowers

CHARACTER Cold
MERIDIANS Lung, Stomach, Large Intestine
ACTIONS Antibacterial, antiviral, hypotensive

Jin yin hua means "gold silver flower" and the herb is used for superficial Wind-Heat conditions as well as internal disorders related to Damp-Heat in the lower *jiao* and Fire Poisons causing swellings especially in the breast, throat, or eyes.

● *Jin yin hua* should be avoided in Deficient and Cold conditions.

● **HOW TO USE** *Jin yin hua* is used with herbs like *jing jie* (schizonepeta) and *bo he* (field mint) for External Wind-Heat or with *huang qin* (baikal skullcap) for feverish conditions. With *jie geng* (balloon flower) and *nui bang zi* (burdock seeds) it is used for pain and swelling in the throat.

Lian qiao forsythia fruits

BOTANICAL NAME *Forsythia suspensa*
TASTE Bitter
CHARACTER Slightly cold
MERIDIANS Lung, Heart, Gall Bladder
ACTIONS Antibacterial, antiemetic, antiparasitic

Lian qiao is effective at clearing External Heat and deeper-seated Fire Poisons causing abscesses, sores, and swellings. It is used for feverish colds with sore throats and headaches, for infections involving swollen neck glands or lymph nodes, and for urinary tract infections.
● Avoid *lian qiao* in diarrhea associated with Deficient Spleen, fevers linked to Deficient *qi* and purulent abscesses.
● **HOW TO USE** For external Heat problems *lian qiao* is often used with *niu bang zi* (burdock seeds), *jing jie* (schizonepeta) and *bo he* (field mint); for internal problems—skin rashes and abscesses—combine with *mu dan pi* (tree peony root bark), *chi shao yao* (red peony), or *xuan shen* (Ningpo figwort root).

HERBS THAT CLEAR SUMMER HEAT

Summer heat is a seasonal disorder typified by fever, irritability, thirst, and diarrhea.

Qing hao sweet wormwood

BOTANICAL NAME *Artemisia annua*
TASTE Bitter
CHARACTER Cold
MERIDIANS Liver, Gall Bladder
ACTIONS Antibacterial, antifungal, antimalarial

Sweet wormwood is regarded by many as a low cost antimalarial remedy. It is used for cooling Blood, clearing fevers associated with Deficient Blood, and reducing Heat associated with Deficient *yin*.
● Avoid in diarrhea or if there are no signs of Heat due to Deficient *yin*.
● **HOW TO USE** *Qing hao* has been used on is own in doses of up to 40g for malaria. It is combined with *sheng di huang* (Chinese foxglove) and *mu dan pi* (tree peony root bark) for Heat associated with Deficient *yin*.

DOWNWARD DRAINING HERBS

Herbs in this group can be described as moist laxatives, purgative and cathartics. They all stimulate or lubricate the gastro-intestinal tract to encourage defecation. Purgatives are used for Interior Excess syndromes including constipation caused by Excess Heat or pathogenic Cold. Moist laxatives lubricate the intestines and are used where constipation is associated with Deficient Blood, *yin*, or *qi*. Cathartics are powerful remedies used where constipation is associated with Stagnation of Fluid or poor water metabolism. They can damage *yin* and *qi* if misused and should only be used by qualified practitioners.

Da huang Chinese rhubarb root

BOTANICAL NAME *Rheum palmatum*
TASTE Bitter
CHARACTER Cold
MERIDIANS Liver, Spleen, Stomach, Large Intestine
ACTIONS Purgative, antibacterial, antifungal, antiparasitic, hypotensive, lowers blood cholesterol levels, cholagogue, diuretic, hemostatic

Rhubarb root is an important herb in the purgative category. It is used for constipation associated with pathogenic Heat, and for dysentery-like disorders related to Damp Heat. It also invigorates Blood and clears Fire Poisons.

● Avoid *da huang* where there are no Heat or Fire symptoms.

● **HOW TO USE** *Da huang* can be used with *rou gou* (cinnamon bark) for constipation or with *huang lian* (Chinese golden thread) and *huang* *qin* (baikal skullcap root) for abdominal bloating associated with Heat or nosebleeds and vomiting blood due to Marauding Hot Blood. It is made into a paste with *shi gao* (gypsum) for burns.

Huo ma ren hemp seeds

BOTANICAL NAME *Cannabis sativa*
TASTE Sweet
CHARACTER Neutral
MERIDIANS Spleen, Stomach, Large Intestine
ACTIONS Laxative, hypotensive

Cannabis seeds are used as a moist laxative in Chinese medicine. They moisten the Intestines and nourish *yin*. Deficient *yin* can be a cause of constipation in the elderly or after feverish illnesses. They also clear Heat and encourage healing of sores so are often added to remedies for ulceration or applied topically.

● Avoid cannabis seeds in diarrhea
● **HOW TO USE** *Huo ma ren* is

combined with *dang gui* (Chinese angelica) for constipation in the elderly or after childbirth. It is combined with herbs such as *jin yin hua* (honeysuckle flowers) and *gan cao* (liquorice) for problems associated with Stomach Heat.

OTHER PURGATIVE HERBS

● *Fan zie ye* (*Cassia angustifolia*): senna leaf is used to clear excess Heat especially in habitual constipation; it should be avoided in pregnancy.
● *Lu hui* (*Aloe vera*): aloe juice purges Heat from the Liver and Large Intestine and is used where symptoms include headache, dizziness, and tinnitus.

Hemp seeds

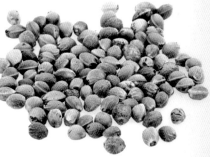

HERBS TO CLEAR DAMPNESS

In Chinese medicine "dampness" can mean excess fluid in the body or suggest a Damp-Heat problem such as "Damp Warm Febrile diseases" or purulent rashes. Herbs used to drain Dampness are diuretic—increasing urination—in conventional medicine.

Fu Ling tuckahoe or Indian bread fungus

BOTANICAL NAME *Poria cocos*
TASTE Sweet, neutral
CHARACTER Neutral
MERIDIANS Lung, Spleen, Heart, Urinary Bladder
ACTIONS Diuretic, sedative, hypoglycemic

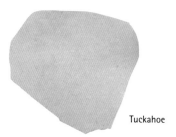

Tuckahoe

Fu ling has been used as a diuretic for Dampness and Phlegm since the days of Shen Nong. While the whole sclerotium is known as *fu ling*, the skin is separated as *fu ling pi* and used as a diuretic while the central part of the sclerotium is *fu shen* used as a calming remedy for the Heart.

● Avoid *fu ling* in excessive urination or prolapse of the urogenital organs.

● **HOW TO USE** *Fu ling* is combined with *gui zhi* (cinnamon twigs) and *bai zhu* (white atractylodes) and *ze xie* (water plantain) for Damp-Heat conditions such as Painful Urinary Dysfunction or with *ban xia* (pinellia) and *chen pi* (tangerine peel) for Congested Fluid syndromes with vomiting and loss of appetite.

Mu tong akebia stems

BOTANICAL NAME *Akebia trifoliata*
TASTE Bitter
CHARACTER Cool
MERIDIANS Heart,
Small Intestine, Urinary
Bladder
ACTIONS Antibacterial,
antifungal, diuretic,
antitumour, anti-
inflammatory, analgesic,
immune stimulant

Fresh akebia
plant

Until the 17th century *mu tong* was generally sourced from akebia species, but in the 1950s the commonest source came from *Aristolochia manshuriensis*, which is rich in aristolochic acid and is now known to cause kidney failure. As such *mu tong* became discredited. Today, akebia is once again being used for *mu tong* as is *Clematis montana*. The herb is mainly used as a diuretic in urinary conditions.

● Avoid in pregnancy or if there is frequent urination.

● **HOW TO USE** *Mu tong* is included in several patent remedies including

long dan xie gan tang (decoction to purge the Liver Fire with gentian), with *huang qi* (milk vetch) and *dang gui* (Chinese angelica) for poor milk flow in breastfeeding associated with Deficient *qi*. It is used with *huai niu xi* (ox knee root) and *hong hua* (safflower) for menstrual problems associated with Congealed Blood.

Several traditional formulae containing *mu tong* have been modified by suppliers to avoid the herb, although as the stems of *Clematis montana* (a common garden climber) make a suitable substitute safe alternatives should be readily available.

Ze xie water plantain rhizome

BOTANICAL NAME A*lisma plantago-aquatica*
TASTE Sweet
CHARACTER Cold
MERIDIANS Kidney, Urinary Bladder
ACTIONS Diuretic, hypotensive, anti-bacterial. hypoglycemic

Water plantain is an effective diuretic used for problems associated with Excess Dampness. It also drains Kidney Fire so is used for Deficient Kidney *yin* associated with excess Heat where symptoms can include dizziness and tinnitus.
● Avoid *ze xie* in seminal emissions associated with Deficient Kidney *yang* or Damp-Cold.

● **HOW TO USE** *Ze xie* is used in *fu ling ze xie tang* (tuckahoe and plantain decoction), which also contains *gui zhi* (cinnamon twigs) and *sheng jiang* (fresh ginger) and is used to clear Dampness in the Stomach; or in *liu wei di huang* (pills of six ingredients with Chinese foxglove) used to strengthen Kidney and Liver *yin*.

Qu mai pinks

BOTANICAL NAME *Dianthus superbus* or *D. chinensis*
TASTE Bitter
CHARACTER Cold
MERIDIANS Heart, Kidney, Small

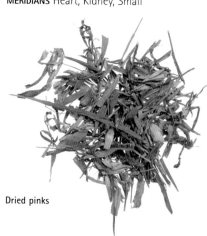

Dried pinks

Intestine, Urinary Bladder
ACTIONS Diuretic, hypotensive,
anti-bacterial

Qu mai is one of the original herbs
listed by Shen Nong. It is used for
constipation as well as to increase
urination. It clears Damp Heat and is
also used for menstrual problems
associated with Congealed Blood.
● Avoid in pregnancy or if there is
Spleen or Kidney Deficiency.
● **HOW TO USE** *Qu mai* is used with
hua shi (talcum) for Heat problems
causing painful urination; with *zhi
zi* (gardenia seeds) where urinary
problems are associated with Damp
Heat in the lower *jiao*; and with
dan shen (Chinese sage) for some
menstrual disorders. It is included
in several patent remedies including
ba zheng san (powder of eight
ingredients to correct urinary
disturbance

OTHER SUBSTANCES TO CLEAR DAMPNESS

● *Hua shi:* talcum is used to clear
Heat from the Urinary Bladder and
is also applied topically for Damp
skin lesions.
● *Deng xin cao* (*Juncus effusus*):
rush pith is used to clear Damp and
Heat from the Heart channel.
● *Bian xu* (*Polygonum aviculare*):
knotgrass is used for Damp Heat in
the Urinary Bladder.
● *Che qian zi* (*Plantago asiatica*):
plantain seed is used for clearing
Damp Heat and for eye problems
associated with Deficient Liver and
Kidney and also to clear Lung Heat
causing coughing.
● *Yi yi ren* (*Coix lachryma-jobi*):
Job's tear seeds are used for various
sorts of edema and are also added
to remedies for Deficient Spleen
to clear Heat and expel Wind-
Dampness.
● *Fang ji* (*Stephania tetranda* or
Aristolochia fangchi): these two
species are differentiated as *han fang
ji* and *guang fang ji* respectively; both
are used to expel Wind Dampness and
encourage urination. *Guang fang ji* is
toxic and should be avoided.

HERBS THAT EXPEL WIND DAMPNESS

These herbs clear Wind Dampness affecting the muscles, joints, bones, tendons, and ligaments which cause "Painful Obstruction" and *bi* syndrome—disorders which conventional medicine may label as arthritis, rheumatism, sciatica, or gout, for example. Painful Obstruction disorders can be linked to Wind, Cold, Damp, or Heat so herbs in this group can vary significantly in character. Many are also tonic remedies for Kidney or Liver associated in the five element model with bones and tendons respectively.

Du huo pubescent angelica root

BOTANICAL NAME *Angelica pubescens*
TASTE Pungent, bitter
CHARACTER Slightly warm
MERIDIANS Kidney, Urinary Bladder
ACTIONS Antirheumatic, analgesic, anti-inflammatory, sedative, hypotensive, nervous stimulant

Du hou is specific for clearing Wind-Damp and relieving pain, especially Wind-Cold-Damp syndromes in the lower part of the body, and is used to combat attack by the external pathogens Wind and Damp so is helpful for superficial syndromes such as colds, rheumatic aches and pains, toothache, and headaches.

● Avoid in *yin* Deficiency and Excess Fire syndromes.

● **HOW TO USE** *Du hou* is one of the main ingredients in *du huo ji sheng tang* (decoction of pubescent angelica and mulberry mistletoe) and is used for arthritic pains and sciatica. It is used with *bo he* (field mint) and *fu ling* (tuckahoe) for external Wind-Cold-Damp disorders.

Cang er zi cocklebur fruit

BOTANICAL NAME *Xanthium strumarium*
TASTE Pungent, slightly bitter
CHARACTER Warm, slightly toxic
MERIDIANS Lung, Liver
ACTIONS Antibacterial, antifungal, antispasmodic, analgesic, antirheumatic

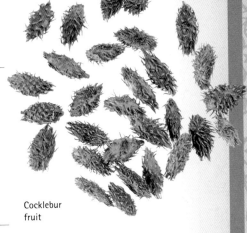

Cocklebur fruit

As well as clearing Wind-Damp, *cang er zi* is said to be helpful for catarrhal conditions such as allergic rhinitis and sinusitis. It also clears external Wind and is used when Wind-Damp causes itching.

● Avoid in headache or Painful Obstruction caused by Deficient Blood.

● **HOW TO USE** *Cang er zi* is combined with herbs such as *xin yi hua* (magnolia flowers), *shi gao* (gypsum), and *huang qin* (baikal skullcap) for acute Wind-Heat syndromes; with *wu wei zi* (schizandra fruits) and *jin ying zi* (rosehips) for allergic rhinitis; and with *jin yin hua* (honeysuckle flowers) for chronic Wind-Heat disorders. With *huang qi* (astragalus root) and *bai zhu* (white atractylodes) it is used as a tonic remedy where *wei qi* is weak.

OTHER HERBS THAT EXPEL WIND DAMPNESS

● *Qin jiao* (*Gentiana macrophylla*): large-leaf gentian root is used for Wind-Damp Painful Obstruction and to moisten the Intestines in constipation.

● *Qi jia pi* (*Eleutherococcus senticosus*): Siberian ginseng root bark is recommended for elderly people who have problems walking and to enhance stamina.

● *Sang zhi* (*Morus alba*): mulberry twigs are used for Wind Dampness causing Painful Obstruction.

HERBS TO CLEAR PHLEGM AND STOP COUGHING

In Chinese medicine Phlegm is not just the sputum coughed up by the lung but a pathological accumulation of thick fluid that can affect other parts of the body especially the Channels, Stomach, and Spleen. If Phlegm stagnates in the Channels it can cause goiter and lymphatic swellings; in the Stomach it can lead to nausea and vomiting, and in the Lungs to coughing and wheezing. Phlegm obstructing the Heart can cause strokes and seizures.

HERBS TO COOL AND TRANSFORM HOT PHLEGM

These herbs are cold and are used to treat coughs and swellings due to Hot Phlegm such as scrofula and goiter. Most are antitussive, expectorant, sedative, and anti-inflammatory.

Zhe bei mu fritillary bulb

BOTANICAL NAME *Fritillaria thunbergii*
TASTE Bitter
CHARACTER Cold

MERIDIANS Lung, Heart
ACTIONS Antitussive, hypotensive, muscle relaxant

Zhe bei mu is used to clear and transform Hot Phlegm that can cause productive coughs. It also combats Heat and is used to reduce swellings including abscesses. Several species of *Fritillaria* are used in Chinese medicine—*chuan bei mu* (*F. cirrhosa*) is also used for cooling and transforming Hot Phlegm. Not as strong as *zhe bei mu*, it is more suitable for non-productive coughs. Both plants are sometimes used together simply as *bei mu*.

● Avoid in Deficient Spleen patterns.

● **HOW TO USE** *Zhe bei mu* is combined with *lian qiao* (forsythia fruits) and *niu bang zi* (burdock seeds) for coughs with thick yellow sputum caused by Wind-Heat. With *xuan shen* (Ningpo figwort root) and *xia ku cao* (self-heal spikes), it is used for Phlegm Fire causing painful swellings and with *yi yi ren* (Job's tear seeds) and other herbs for lung abscesses.

OTHER HERBS TO COOL AND TRANSFORM PHLEGM

● *Qian hu* (*Peucedanum praeruptorum*): peucedanum root is used to direct *qi* downward as well as clear Phlegm. It is also used for pathogenic Wind conditions.

● *Gua lou* (*Trichosanthes kirilowii*): snakegourd fruit is used to moisten the Lung, resolve Phlegm, and invigorate Lung *qi*.

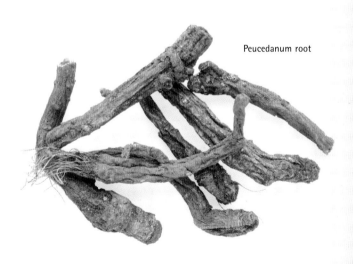

Peucedanum root

WARM HERBS TO TRANSFORM COLD PHLEGM

These herbs are warm and can be toxic so care is needed in their preparation and use.

Ban xia pinellia tuber

BOTANICAL NAME *Pinellia ternata*
TASTE Pungent
CHARACTER Warm, toxic
MERIDIANS Lung, Spleen, Stomach
ACTIONS Antiemetic, antitussive, expectorant, lowers blood cholesterol levels, antidote for strychnine poisoning

Ban xia is effective for drying Dampness and transforming Phlegm. It also reverses the flow of rebellious *qi*, responsible for certain types of vomiting and productive coughs. *Ban xia* clears Damp Phlegm from the Stomach, and dispels nodules and discomfort in the chest. It is usually soaked in tea or vinegar before use to reduce its toxicity.
● Avoid in bleeding, Deficient *yin* coughs, pregnancy, and Phlegm-Heat conditions. Long-term over-use can lead to loss of taste and numbness in the mouth and throat.
● **HOW TO USE** *Ban xia* is used in numerous remedies for Phlegm related disorders. With *gan jiang* (dried ginger) it subdues Rebellious *qi* caused by *yang* Deficiency and clears Cold; with *chen pi* (tangerine peel) and other herbs it is used for productive coughs caused by Damp Phlegm Obstruction or Deficient Spleen *qi*.

Jie geng balloon flower root

BOTANICAL NAME *Platycodon grandiflorum*
TASTE Pungent, bitter
CHARACTER Neutral
MERIDIANS Lung
ACTIONS Anti-fungal, anti-bacterial, expectorant, hypoglycemic, reduces cholesterol levels

Jie geng helps circulate Lung *qi* and clear Phlegm, especially when caused by Wind-Heat or Wind-Cold; it is also useful for sore throats and

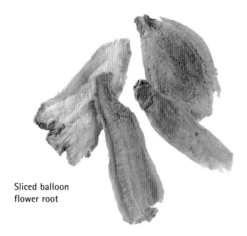

Sliced balloon
flower root

laryngitis associated with external
Heat, Deficient *yin* with Heat signs
and Hot Phlegm. It is one of the
directional herbs focusing the
remedy upward to the upper
part of the body.

● Avoid in tuberculosis or coughing
up blood

● **HOW TO USE** *Jie geng* is used with
gan cao (liquorice) for swellings and
pain in the throat caused by Wind-
Heat and with *zi su ye* (perilla leaf)
for productive coughs due to
external Wind-Cold. It is combined
with *ban xia* (pinellia) for coughs
caused by Damp Phlegm.

OTHER WARM HERBS TO TRANSFORM COLD PHLEGM

● *Xuan fu hua* (*Inula brittanica*):
Japanese elecampane flower head is
also a directional remedy correcting
the upward flow of Lung and
Stomach *qi* that may cause coughs;
it resolves Phlegm Stagnation in
the Lung.

● *Bai jie zi* (*Brassica alba*): white
mustard seed helps to warm Lung *qi*
and ease pain caused by Cold Phlegm
in the Channels. It is used for both
pleurisy and joint pain.

HERBS TO RELIEVE COUGHING AND WHEEZING

These herbs provide symptomatic relief so are always combined with appropriate remedies to treat the underlying cause; they are generally antitussive, expectorant, and antibiotic.

Xing ren bitter apricot seeds

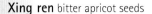

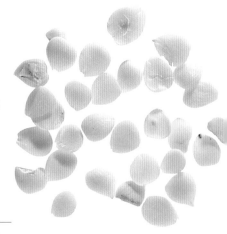

Processed bitter apricot seeds

BOTANICAL NAME *Prunus armeniaca*
TASTE Bitter
CHARACTER Slightly warm, slightly toxic
MERIDIANS Lung, Large Intestine
actions Antitussive, antiasthmatic, antibacterial, antiparasitic, analgesic

Xing ren is used where symptoms include coughing caused by Cold or Heat problems. The seeds are effective for dry coughs and also to moisten the intestines in constipation. *Xing ren* is generally steamed or baked before use to reduce toxicity.

● Avoid in coughs caused by Deficient *yin*. Apricot seeds contain hydrocyanic acid and high doses can be toxic.

● **HOW TO USE** *Xing ren* is used with herbs such as *huo ma ren* (hemp seed) for constipation caused by dryness or Deficient *qi* and with *shi gao* (gypsum), *zhe bei mu* (fritillary bulb), and *gua lou zi* (snakegourd fruit) for External Wind-Heat problems with cough producing thick, yellow sputum.

Sang bai pi mulberry root bark

BOTANICAL NAME *Morus alba*
TASTE Sweet
CHARACTER Cold
MERIDIANS Lung, Spleen
ACTIONS Various parts of the mulberry are analgesic, antiasthmatic, antibacterial, antitussive, diaphoretic, diuretic, expectorant, hypotensive, hypoglycemic, and sedative

Sang bai pi is largely used as a cough remedy for Heat in the Lung and asthma. Mulberry twigs (*sang zhi*) are used for rheumatic pains and spasms while the leaf (*sang ye*) is for Wind and Heat and the fruits (*sang shen*) nourish the Blood.

● Avoid the root bark in Cold conditions and Deficient Lung.

● **HOW TO USE** *Sang bai pi* is also a diuretic and used with herbs such as *fu ling pi* (tuckahoe skin), and *chen pi* (tangerine peel) for edema caused by Fluid imbalance associated with Deficient Spleen *qi*.

OTHER HERBS TO RELIEVE COUGHING AND WHEEZING

● *Kuan dong hua* (*Tussilago farfara*): coltsfoot flower redirects *qi* downward and stops coughing.

● *Zi su zi* (*Perilla frutescens*): perilla seed redirects *qi* downward, dissolves Phlegm, and also moistens the Intestines in constipation caused by Dryness.

● *Zi wan* (*Aster tartaricus*): purple aster root stops a wide range of coughs epecially where Cold and copious sputum are involved.

Sliced mulberry root bark

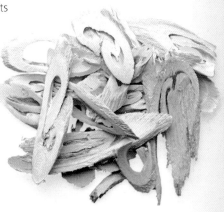

AROMATIC HERBS

AROMATIC HERBS TO TRANSFORM DAMPNESS

These herbs are used to clear Dampness associated with Stagnation of the middle *jiao* with nausea, vomiting, abdominal distention, and loss of appetite. They are all pungent and dry and used with caution if there is any *yin* Deficiency.

Huo xiang patchouli or giant hyssop

BOTANICAL NAMES *Pogostemon cablin* or *Agastache rugosa*
TASTE Pungent
CHARACTER Slightly warm
MERIDIANS Lung, Spleen, Stomach

ACTIONS Antibacterial, antifungal, diaphoretic, digestive tonic

Huo xiang can be two different plants. Both patchouli (*Pogostemon cablin*) and giant hyssop (*Agastache rugosa*) are used medicinally as *huo xiang*. As well as clearing Damp it dispels Cold and harmonizes the middle *jiao*.

● Avoid in fevers and Interior Heat syndromes.

● **HOW TO USE** *Hou xiang* is included in *huo xiang zheng qi san* (powder for dispelling turbidity with giant hyssop), which is used to clear Dampness from Spleen and Stomach. For acute diarrhea associated with Heat and Dampness, it is used with such herbs as *huang qin* (baikal skullcap) and *lian qiao* (forsythia fruits).

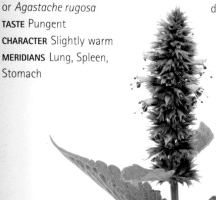

Giant hyssop flower head

Cang zhu Grey atractylodes
rhizome

BOTANICAL NAME *Atractylodes chinensis*
TASTE Pungent, bitter
CHARACTER Warm
MERIDIANS Spleen, Stomach
ACTIONS Carminative, diaphoretic, increases excretion of sodium and potassium salts, although it is not diuretic

Cang zhu is used for Dampness in the lower *jiao*, Wind-Dampness associated with painful obstruction, Dampness causing Spleen problems and also for external problems associated with Wind-Cold-Damp.

● Avoid in *qi* or *yin* Deficiency associated with Interior Heat.
● **HOW TO USE** *Cang zhu* is used for digestive problems associated with Damp Cold stagnating in the Spleen with herbs such as *hou po* (magnolia bark) and *chen pi* (tangerine peel). *Cang zhu* is a traditional remedy for night blindness and cataracts when combined with *hei zhi ma* (sesame seeds) and other herbs.

OTHER AROMATIC HERBS TO TRANSFORM DAMPNESS

● *Huo po* (*Magnolia officinalis*): magnolia bark is used to move *qi*, warm and transform Phlegm, and clear Stagnation. It is used for both digestive and respiratory problems.
● *Sha ren* (*Amomum xanthoides*): grains of paradise or bastard cardamomis are used to move *qi*, strengthen the Stomach and calm the fetus in morning sickness.

AROMATIC HERBS TO OPEN ORIFICES

These are mainly used for "Locked-in Syndrome" (bì zhèng) following strokes that lead to coma and rigid limbs. They stimulate the central nervous system and can drain congenital *qi* so should only be used for a short time.

● *Bing pian* (*Dryobalanops aromatica*): borneol resin is used for fainting and convulsions
● *Shi chang pu*, also called *chang pu* (*Acorus gramineus*): sweetflag rhizome clears Phlegm that causes deafness, dizziness, and dulled senses.

HERBS TO RELIEVE FOOD STAGNATION

Symptoms of food stagnation include abdominal distention and nausea with a preference for either hot or cold foods depending on whether the stagnation is a Cold disorder or a Hot one. The herbs in this group are mainly digestive stimulants.

Shan zha Chinese hawthorn berries

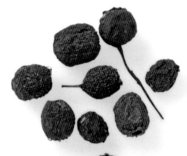

Fresh Chinese
hawthorn berries

BOTANICAL NAME *Crataegus pinnatifida*
TASTE Sour, sweet
CHARACTER Slightly warm
MERIDIANS Spleen, Stomach, Liver
ACTIONS Antibacterial, hypotensive, peripheral vasodilator, cardiac tonic, lowers cholesterol levels

As well as easing food stagnation, *shan zha* is used to invigorate Blood circulation and generally improve digestion.

● Avoid or use *shan zha* cautiously in cases of Deficient Spleen and Stomach and if there is acid regurgitation.

● **HOW TO USE** *Shan zha* is traditionally combined with *mai ya* (barley sprouts) and *shen qu* (medicated leaves) for food stagnation. *Shan zha* is also used with remedies like *dang gui* (Chinese angelica) for Congealed Blood that can cause some menstrual pain.

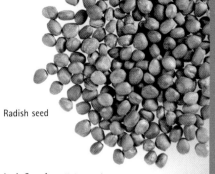
Radish seed

Mai ya barley sprouts

BOTANICAL NAME *Hordium vulgare*
TASTE Sweet
CHARACTER Slightly warm
MERIDIANS Spleen, Stomach
ACTIONS Contains enzymes and vitamin B, which aid digestion

While barley sprouts are used in decoctions and powders with other herbs, they are also eaten either raw or toasted to clear Food Stagnation or strengthen the Spleen. They also reduce milk flow and are traditionally taken for weaning, when they should be stir fried. *Mai ya* can also be given to babies to treat milk regurgitation and dyspepsia in babies.

● Avoid when breastfeeding.

● **HOW TO USE** *Mai ya* is combined with a number of herbs including *fu ling* (tuckahoe) and *bai zhu* (white atractylodes) in *jian pi wan* (strengthening the Spleen pills) used for Spleen and Stomach Deficiency with Food Stagnation. It is used with *gan jiang* (dried ginger) for indigestion associated with Stomach Deficiency.

Lai fu zi radish seed

BOTANICAL NAME *Raphanus sativa*
TASTE Pungent, sweet
CHARACTER Neutral
MERIDIANS Lung, Spleen, Stomach
ACTIONS Antimicrobial, antifungal

As well as dissolving Food Stagnation, *lai fu zi* causes *qi* to descend and transforms Phlegm so is also used in chronic coughs.

● Use cautiously if there is Deficient *yin*.

● **HOW TO USE** *Lai fu zi* is combined with *shan zha* (hawthorn berries) or *chen pi* (tangerine peel) for Food Stagnation; and is used with *ban xia* (pinellia), *xing ren* (bitter apricot seeds), or *zi su zi* (perilla seeds) where there is chronic coughing that may be associated with Damp Phlegm or excess Heat.

HERBS TO WARM THE INTERIOR AND EXPEL COLD

Interior Cold can be caused by pathogenic Cold invading the body or by internally generated Cold, sometimes associated with shock or Deficiency syndromes. Herbs to expel Cold generally warm the Spleen and Kidney and are often used with herbs that tonify *yang* or *qi*.

Wu zhu yu evodia berries

BOTANICAL NAME *Evodia rutacarpa*
TASTE Pungent, bitter
CHARACTER Hot, slightly toxic
MERIDIANS Spleen, Stomach, Liver, Kidney
ACTIONS Antibacterial, antiparasitic, analgesic, raises body temperature, respiratory stimulant, uterine stimulant

Wu zhu yu warms the Spleen and Stomach and also reverses the flow of *qi* associated with vomiting and acid regurgitation.
● Avoid in *yin* Deficiency and Excess Fire.

● HOW TO USE *Wu zhu yu* is is traditionally mixed with liquorice water to reduce its toxicity or cooked with ginger to relieve abdominal pain caused by Cold. When stir-baked (stir-fried without oil) it is used to reverse the upward flow of Stomach and Liver *qi*.

Ding xiang cloves

BOTANICAL NAME *Syzygium aromaticum*
TASTE Pungent
CHARACTER Warm
MERIDIANS Spleen, Stomach, Kidney
ACTIONS Carminative, antiemetic,

antibacterial, analgesic, anti-inflammatory, causes uterine contractions

---

Cloves are used in Chinese medicine to warm the *san jiao* and Kidneys and also to cause Rebellious *qi* to descend. The herb also strengthens Kidney.

● Avoid in *yin* Deficiency and Heat syndromes.

● **HOW TO USE** Cloves are used with *Wu zhu yu* (evodia berries) for abdominal pain and vomiting associated with Cold Stomach and with *rou gui* (cinnamon bark) for impotence associated with deficient Kidneys.

OTHER HERBS TO WARM THE INTERIOR AND EXPEL COLD

● *Fu zi* (*Aconite carmichaeli*): Szechuan aconite is an extremely toxic plant and not one for lay use. It is prepared by cooking in ginger to reduce its toxicity and is used for both Cold conditions and to restore and strengthen *yang*, especially affecting Spleen and Kidney.

● *Gan jiang* (*Zingiber officinale*): dry ginger has a tonic action and enters the Kidney meridian, where it is used to replenish *yang*, expel Cold and warm Spleen and Stomach.

● *Rou gui* (*Cinnamomum cassia*): cinnamon bark, as well as clearing Interior Cold, is used to warm and tonify the Kidneys.

● *Xiao hui xiang* (*Foeniculum vulgare*): fennel seeds regulate *qi* and warm the *san jiao*; as in the West they are mainly used for digestive problems.

● *Gao liang jiang* (*Alpinia officinarum*): galangal rhizome is used to warm the middle *jiao* and relieve pain.

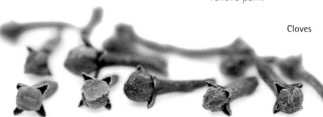

Cloves

HERBS TO REGULATE QI

These herbs can be divided into two groups—herbs to move Stagnant *qi* and tonic herbs used in Deficient *qi* disorders.

HERBS TO MOVE STAGNANT *QI*

Stagnant qi conditions are characterized by pain in the organs affected. These herbs tend to be dry so prolonged use can damage *yin*.

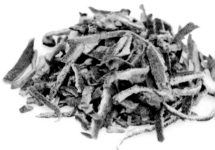

Shredded tangerine peel

Chen pi tangerine peel

BOTANICAL NAME *Citrus reticulata*
TASTE Pungent, bitter
CHARACTER Warm
MERIDIANS Lung, Spleen, Stomach
ACTIONS Anti-asthmatic, anti-inflammatory, carminative, digestive stimulant, expectorant, circulatory stimulant; trials have shown it to be effective for acute mastitis

Chen pi is the ripe peel from tangerines or mandarins while *qing pi* is the green peel from the same unripe fruit and enters Liver and Gall Bladder meridians.

● Avoid in cases of coughing up blood or if there is no sign of Damp/Phlegm stagnation.

● **HOW TO USE** *Chen pi* is a widely used ingredient in remedies for coughing and nausea where disordered *qi* is to blame. For problems associated with Stagnant Spleen and Stomach *qi*, it is used in *ping wei san* (calm Stomach powder). *Chen pi* improves with storage.

Xiang fu Nutgrass tuber

BOTANICAL NAME *Cyperus rotundus*
TASTE Pungent, slightly bitter
CHARACTER Neutral
MERIDIANS Liver, Stomach
ACTIONS Analgesic, antibacterial, antispasmodic for the uterus

Xiang fu helps to circulate *qi* especially where Constrained Liver *qi* is the problem, and is used for menstrual problems, normalizing the cycle and easing period pains. It is prepared with vinegar to enhance its painkilling effect or salt to help moisten Blood and Fluids.

● Avoid in Heat syndromes associated with *yin* Deficiency.

● **HOW TO USE** *Xiang fu* is used with *bai zhu* (white atractylodes) and *ban xia* (pinellia) for Spleen or Stomach Deficiency and added to mixtures like *xiang sha ping wei san* (nutgrass and grains of paradise powder to calm the Stomach). It is used with *dang gui* (Chinese angelica) for menstrual irregularities.

OTHER HERBS TO MOVE STAGNANT QI

● *Mu xiang* (*Saussurea kappa* or *Vladimiria souliei*): costus root is mainly used for problems with Spleen or Stomach *qi*.

● *Tan xiang* (*Santalum album*): sandalwood is used for Stagnant Spleen or Stomach *qi*.

● *Zhi shi* and *zhi ke* (*Citrus aurantium*): the immature fruit of the bitter (Seville) orange is used to break up Stagnant *qi* and direct it downward.

● *Xie bai* (*Allium macrostemon*): Chinese chive is used to move *qi* and Blood and also dissipate Cold Phlegm; it directs *qi* downward.

● *Da fu pi* (*Areca catechu*): betel husk is used for Spleen and Stomach *qi* Stagnation.

Nutgrass tuber

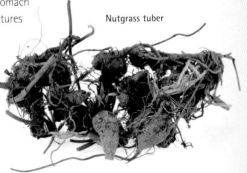

HERBS TO TONIFY *QI*

These herbs are used in *qi* Deficiency where particular organs or functions are weak—most commonly Lungs or Spleen. They are sweet and rich and over-use can lead to sensations of heat or fullness in the upper body. It is best to avoid taking tonic herbs when suffering from infectious diseases.

Ren shen Korean ginseng root

BOTANICAL NAME *Panax ginseng*
TASTE Sweet, slightly bitter
CHARACTER Warm
MERIDIANS Spleen, Lung, Heart
ACTIONS Tonic, stimulant, reduces blood sugar and cholesterol levels, immunostimulant

---

Korean or red ginseng is the best known of China's many tonic herbs. It is used to replenish and tonify *qi*, to generate body fluids and to combat fatigue.

● Avoid in Heat conditions.

● **HOW TO USE** *Ren shen* is a powerful *qi* tonic and is included in many formulae. With *bai zhu* (white atractylodes) it is used for Deficient Spleen and Stomach *qi*; with *fu ling* (tuckahoe) for Deficient Heart and Spleen; or with *wu wei zi* (schizandra) for Deficient *qi* and *yin* conditions.

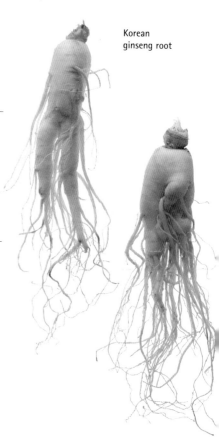

Korean
ginseng root

Huang qi milk vetch root

BOTANICAL NAME *Astragalus membranaceus*
TASTE Sweet
CHARACTER Slightly warm
MERIDIANS Spleen, Lung
ACTIONS Antispasmodic, diuretic, cholagogue, antibacterial, hypoglycemic, nervous stimulant, hypotensive, immune stimulant

Huang qi helps to strengthen defence energy, so is believed to boost the immune system. It also encourages wound healing and helps regulate water metabolism, as well as tonifying *qi* and Blood.
● Avoid in Excess syndromes or if there is Deficient *yin*.
● **HOW TO USE** *Huang qi* is included with *ren shen* (Korean ginseng) and *bai zhu* (white atractylodes) in *bu zhong yi qi tang* used to combat Spleen and Stomach Deficiency or with *dang gui* (Chinese angelica) to nourish blood in anemia and Blood Deficiency.

Bai zhu White atractylodes rhizome

BOTANICAL NAME *Atractylodes macrocephala*
TASTE Sweet, bitter
CHARACTER Warm
MERIDIANS Spleen, Stomach
ACTIONS Antibacterial, anticoagulant, digestive stimulant, diuretic, hypoglycemic

Bai zhu tonifies the Spleen and dispels Dampness so tends to be used where symptoms include poor appetite, indigestion, chronic diarrhea, and abdominal fullness. It can also help to boost the *wei qi* to increase resistance in Exterior syndromes.
● Avoid in *yin* Deficiency characterized by extreme thirst.
● **HOW TO USE** *Bai zhu* is included in the famous energy-giving *si jun zi tang* (four noble ingredients decoction) with *ren shen* (Korean ginseng), *fu ling* (tuckahoe), and *gan cao* (liquorice).

Da zao and hong zao Chinese dates

BOTANICAL NAME *Ziziphus vulgaris* var. *jujuba*
TASTE Sweet
CHARACTER Warm
MERIDIANS Spleen, Stomach
ACTIONS Nutrient, protects against liver damage

Da zao and *hong zao* are from the same kind of fruit—when blanched slightly in boiling water and dried under the sun, it is *hong zao* (red jujube), and when the fruit is blanched in boiling water and baked until the skin become black and shiny it is called *da zao* (large jujube). Both nourish the Blood

Chinese red dates

(*hong zao* rather more effectively) and calm the Spirit.

● Avoid in cases of Excess Dampness, Food Stagnation or Phlegm.

● **HOW TO USE** *Da zao* is often combined with harsh cathartic herbs to modify their action and prevent injury to Stomach and Spleen. Chinese dates also "calm the Spirit" so are used for symptoms associated with Deficient Heart syndromes.

Gan cao liquorice root

BOTANICAL NAME *Glycyrrhiza uralensis*
TASTE Sweet
CHARACTER Neutral (raw) or warm (prepared)
MERIDIANS Heart, Lung, Spleen, Stomach
ACTIONS Antibacterial, antitussive, anti-inflammatory, antispasmodic, antiallergenic, hypotensive, steroidal action, cholagogue

Gan cao is used invigorate *qi*, tonify the Spleen, moisten the Lungs to stop coughing and wheezing, and also to clear Heat and

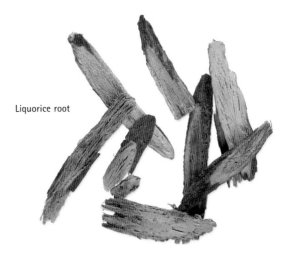

Liquorice root

Fire Poisons. It is often added to prescriptions to harmonize the action of other herbs. Liquorice is sometimes prepared by stir-frying with honey or toasting, in which case it is called *zhi gan cao*.

● Avoid in excess Dampness, nausea or vomiting.

● **HOW TO USE** *Gan cao* is used with *dang shen* (bellflower root) for Deficient Spleen with *gui zhi* (cinnamon twigs) added where there is deficient Heart *qi*. It is used with *bai shao yao* (white peony) for Liver Blood problems associated with pain in the abdomen or with *chen pi* (tangerine peel) and *ban xia* (pinellia) in *er chen tang* (decoction of two old herbs) used to transform and clear Phlegm in chronic bronchitis or gastritis.

OTHER HERBS TO TONIFY QI

● *Dang shen* (*Codonopsis pilosula*): bellflower root is an important tonic that is more *yin* in character than *ren shen* (Korean ginseng) and is traditionally taken by nursing mothers. It is included in *ba zhen tang* (eight treasures decoction) for Deficient *qi* and Blood.

● *Shan yao* (*Dioscorea opposita*): Chinese yam root is used to tonify *qi* of Spleen and Stomach but also nourishes Lung and Kidney.

HERBS TO REGULATE THE BLOOD

Herbs to regulate Blood come into three general categories: those to stop bleeding; those to invigorate the Blood (used in cases of Stagnant or Congealed Blood); and those that tonify the Blood (used when Blood is Deficient).

HERBS TO STOP BLEEDING

Used for a range of conditions ranging from nosebleeds and coughing up blood-streaked sputum to heavy menstrual periods and blood in the urine. They are generally combined with herbs appropriate for the underlying condition.

San qi notoginseng or pseudoginseng root

BOTANICAL NAME *Panax pseudoginseng*
TASTE Sweet, slightly bitter
CHARACTER Warm
MERIDIANS Liver, Stomach

ACTIONS Antibacterial, anti-inflammatory, cardiotonic, circulatory, stimulant, diuretic, hemostatic, hypoglycemic, peripheral vasodilator

San qi (also known as *tian qi*) is used for bleeding associated with Congealed Blood—both internally and

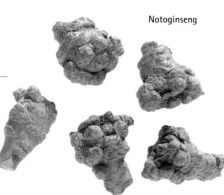

Notoginseng

externally—and will also reduce swelling and relieve pain so is often used for traumatic injuries. It helps to encourage Blood circulation so is also used for chest and abdominal pain.

Artemisia vulgaris var. indica

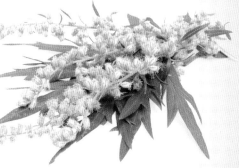

● Avoid *san qi* in pregnancy and only use with caution in Deficient Blood syndromes.

● **HOW TO USE** *San qi* is used by itself in *yun nan bai yao* (Yunnan white remedy) for a wide range of bleeding disorders. It is used in patent remedies such as *san qi shang yao pian* (notoginseng and peony pills), to ease pain in sprains and tendon injuries.

OTHER HERBS TO STOP BLEEDING

● *Pu huang* (*Typha latifolia* and other species): bullrush pollen is used to stop bleeding from external traumatic injuries as well as encouraging Blood circulation and dispelling Congealed Blood.

● *Ai ye* (*Artemisia vulgaris* var. *indica*): mugwort leaf is used in moxibustion but also warms the meridians and stops bleeding. It is included in *jiao ai tang* (donkey hide and mugwort decoction) which is a popular remedy to calm the fetus in threatened miscarriage.

● *Bai ji* (*Bletilla striata*): bletilla rhizome is used for bleeding from the Lungs and Stomach and also reduces swellings and encourages healing.

● *Ce bai ye* (*Biota orientalis*): arborvitae twigs cool the Blood and relieve coughs; they are used for many bleeding disorders including bleeding gums and uterine bleeding.

HERBS TO INVIGORATE THE BLOOD

These herbs are used for problems associated with Stagnant or Congealed Blood that may cause pain, abscesses or ulcers, or Abdominal Swellings, such as tumours (zhēng jiǎ) and cysts.

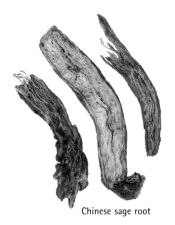

Chinese sage root

Dan shen Chinese sage root

BOTANICAL NAME *Salvia miltiorrhiza*
TASTE Bitter
CHARACTER Slightly cold
MERIDIANS Heart, Liver, Pericardium
ACTIONS Anticoagulant, antibacterial, immune stimulant, circulatory stimulant, peripheral vasodilator, promotes tissue repair, sedative, lowers blood cholesterol, hypoglycemic

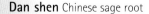

As well as invigorating Blood and dispersing congealed Blood, *dan shen* clears Heat and "calms the Spirit." Modern studies have shown it to be effective for angina pectoris and problems associated with cerebral circulation.

● Avoid if there is no Blood Stagnation.

● **HOW TO USE** *Dan shen* is used with *dang gui* (Chinese angelica) for menstrual problems or with *mu dan pi* (tree peony bark) and *sheng di huang* (Chinese foxglove) for Warm-Febrile diseases.

Chi shao yao red peony root

BOTANICAL NAME *Paeonia lactiflora*
TASTE Sour, bitter
CHARACTER Slightly cold
MERIDIANS Liver, Spleen
ACTIONS Antibacterial, anticoagulant, anti-inflammatory, immune stimulant, lowers blood cholesterol, peripheral

vasodilator, hypoglycemic, sedative, stimulates tissue repair, improves microcirculation

Red peony is used to clear Blood Stagnation, especially where symptoms include period pain, menstrual irregularities or Abdominal Swellings. It is also cooling for Heat in the Blood, especially in fevers and skin conditions, and clears Liver Fire.

● Avoid if there is no evidence of Blood Stagnation.

● **HOW TO USE** *Chi shao yao* is used with *ju hua* (chrysanthemum flowers) and *huang qin* (baikal skullcap) and other herbs for red, swollen eyes, or with *xiang fu* (nutgrass tuber) for period pain or Abdominal Swellings.

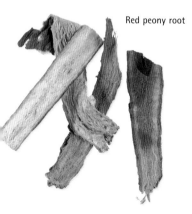

Red peony root

OTHER SUBSTANCES TO INVIGORATE THE BLOOD

● *Huai nu xi* (*Achyranthis bidentata*): ox knee root is used to clear Damp Heat in the lower *jiao* and descend the flow of Blood caused by Deficient *yin* with ascending Fire.

● *Chuan xiong* (*Ligusticum wallichii*): Szechuan lovage root expels Wind, moves *qi* upward, relieves pain, dizziness, and headaches.

● *Yan hu suo* (*Corydalis yanhusuo*): corydalis rhizome is used for pain caused by Congealed Blood such as period pain; it also moves *qi*.

● *Tao ren* (*Prunus persica*): peach seed is used to break up Congealed Blood mainly in menstrual and abdominal problems and to moisten the intestines.

● *Hong hua* (*Carthamis tinctorius*): safflower is used for Congealed Blood in gynecological disorders.

● *Wu ling zhi* (*Trogopterus xanthipes*): flying squirrel droppings are used for Congealed Blood in gynecological disorders.

● *Mo yao* (*Commiphora myrrha*): myrrh also dispels Congealed Blood and promotes healing.

HERBS TO TONIFY THE BLOOD

These herbs are used for Deficient Blood syndromes and are said to "nourish the Blood." Typical symptoms include pale face and lips, dizziness, palpitations, dry skin, and lethargy, associated with iron-deficient anemia in Western medicine.

He shou wu fleeceflower root

BOTANICAL NAME *Polygonum multiflorum*
TASTE Sweet, bitter, astringent
CHARACTER Slightly warm
MERIDIANS Liver, Kidney
ACTIONS Antibacterial, cardiotonic, hormonal action, hyperglycemic, laxative, liver stimulant, reduces blood cholesterol

Fleeceflower root

He shou wu is sometimes sold as *fo ti* (its Cantonese name). It is specific for strengthening Kidney essence so is a valuable menopausal remedy. It is also a moist laxative, detoxifies Fire Poisons causing carbuncles and boils, and expels External Wind by nourishing the Blood.

● Avoid in diarrhea associated with Phlegm or Deficient Spleen.

● **HOW TO USE** *He shou wu* is combined with *xuan shen* (figwort root) and *lian qiao* (forsythia fruits) for abscesses and "Poisonous

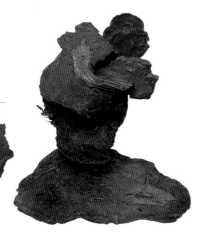

Swellings" or with *gou qi zi* (wolfberry fruit) and *bu gu zi* (scuffy pea) for symptoms of premature ageing associated with deficient Liver and Kidney.

Dang gui Chinese angelica root

BOTANICAL NAME *Angelica polyphorma* var. *sinensis*
TASTE Sweet, pungent
CHARACTER Warm
MERIDIANS Liver, Heart, Spleen
ACTIONS Antibacterial, analgesic, anti-inflammatory, circulatory stimulant, reduces blood cholesterol levels, liver tonic, sedative, uterine stimulant, rich in folic acid and vitamin B12

Dang gui is also sold as *tang kwai* or *dong qui* in tinctures, tablets and powders, and is used to nourish and invigorate the Blood as well as ease pain from Congealed or Stagnant Blood. It is also a moist laxative used for constipation in the elderly.
● Avoid in pregnancy, diarrhea, or abdominal fullness.

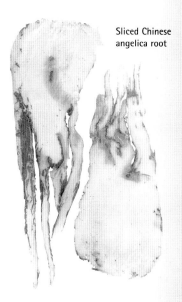

Sliced Chinese angelica root

● **HOW TO USE** *Dang gui* is sometimes combined with *huang qi* (milk vetch root) for debility and fatigue associated with Deficient Blood or with *sheng jiang* (fresh ginger) for pain after childbirth. It is included in numerous classic formulae including *dang gui si ni tang* (Chinese angelica decoction for frigid extremities) also containing *gui zhi* (cinnamon twigs), and *bai shao yao* (white peony), used to disperse Cold and nourish the Blood.

Bai shao yao white peony root

BOTANICAL NAME *Paeonia lactiflora*
TASTE Sour, bitter
CHARACTER Slightly cold
MERIDIANS Liver, Spleen
ACTIONS Antibacterial, anti-inflammatory, antispasmodic, diuretic, sedative, hypotensive, analgesic

Bai shao yao is used to nourish the Blood in Deficient Blood syndromes, it also calms the Liver and relieves pain associated with Constrained Liver *qi* or disharmony between Liver and Spleen. It is also used for Deficient *yin* problems and some Wind Cold syndromes.
● Avoid in diarrhea and abdominal coldness.
● **HOW TO USE** *Bai shao yao* is used with *chai hu* (thorowax root) and *zhi shi* (bitter orange) to calm Liver *qi* and regulate the Spleen; or with *gui zhi* (cinnamon twigs), *sheng jiang* (fresh ginger) and other herbs in *xiao jian zhong tang* (minor decoction to restore the middle *jiao*) for abdominal pain associated with

san jiao weakness. With *gan cao* (liquorice) it is used to nourish the Liver and ease muscle cramps associated with Deficient Blood.

Gou qi zi wolfberry fruits

BOTANICAL NAME *Lycium barbarum* or *L. chinense*
TASTE Sweet
CHARACTER Neutral
MERIDIANS Liver, Kidney
ACTIONS Hypotensive, hypoglycemic, immune stimulant, liver tonic and restorative, lowers blood cholesterol levels

Wolfberry fruits are used to nourish and tonify Liver and Kidney, and said to "brighten the eyes," where Deficient Liver and Kidney is associated with blurred vision, dizziness and eyesight problems. In recent years the berries have gained in popularity as a health food under the name of goji berries.
● Avoid in cases of Excess Heat, and Spleen Deficiency with Dampness.
● **HOW TO USE** *Gou qi zi* is used with

shu di huang (prepared Chinese foxglove) and other herbs for dizziness, tinnitus, impotence, and weakness associated with Deficient *yin* and Blood or with *ju hua* (chrysanthemum flowers) where Deficiency symptoms include tinnitus, headache, and eyesight problems.

OTHER HERBS TO TONIFY THE BLOOD

● *Shu di huang* (*Rehmannia glutinosa*): prepared Chinese foxglove root is the most widely used herb in this group, is slightly warm and as well as nourishing Blood, regulates menstrual flow and replenishes the vital essence of the Kidney.

● *Long yan rou* also called *gui yuan rou* (*Dimocarpus longan*): longan fruit flesh is used to tonify Heart and Spleen, nourish Blood and calm the Spirit and used for insomnia, palpitations, and dizziness.

● *Sang shen* (*Morus alba*): mulberry fruits nourish Blood and Liver and Kidney *yin*; also used for dizziness, insomnia, and premature graying of the hair.

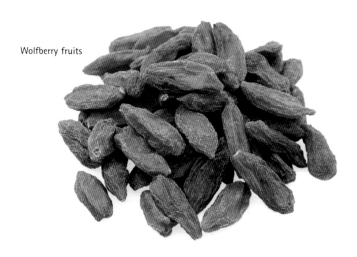

Wolfberry fruits

ASTRINGENT HERBS

These are used for treating conditions involving some sort of Excess discharge—such as diarrhea, excess sweating, frequent urination, or prolapse of the womb or rectum. All these herbs contain large amounts of tannin, which may explain their action.

Shan zhu yu dogwood fruits

BOTANICAL NAME *Cornus officinalis*
TASTE Sour
CHARACTER Warm
MERIDIANS Liver, Kidney
ACTIONS Antibacterial, antifungal, diuretic, hypotensive, styptic

Shan zhu yu stops bleeding so is often used for excessive menstrual bleeding. It helps replenish Liver and Kidney essence so is helpful where symptoms include aching back and knees, vertigo, frequent urination, and sweating.
● Avoid *shan zhu yu* in Fire symptoms and Deficiency Kidney *yang*; it should not be combined with *jie geng* (balloon flower root) or *fang feng* (siler).

● **HOW TO USE** *Shan zhu yu* is combined with *shu di huang* (prepared Chinese foxglove) and *fu ling* (tuckahoe) in *liu wei di huang wan* (six ingredients Chinese foxglove pill) used to nourish Liver and Kidney *yin*. With *huang qi* (milk vetch) and *dang shen* (bellflower root) it is used for spontaneous sweating associated with *yang* or *qi* Deficiency and with *bai shao yao* (white peony) for excessive uterine bleeding.

Dogwood fruits

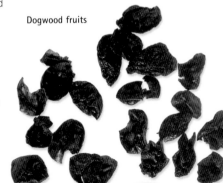

Wu wei zi schizandra fruits

BOTANICAL NAME *Schisandra chinensis*
TASTE Sour
CHARACTER Warm
MERIDIANS Lung, Heart, Kidney
ACTIONS Antibacterial, astringent, aphrodisiac, circulatory stimulant, digestive stimulant, expectorant, hypotensive, sedative, tonic, uterine stimulant

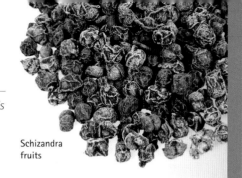

Schizandra fruits

Wu wei zi is used to replenish *qi*, especially Lung *qi*, tonify the Kidney and Heart, calm the Spirit, and control excessive sweating. It is used for a condition sometimes called "cock-crow diarrhea" associated with Spleen and Kidney Deficiency.

● Avoid in cases of Internal Heat and superficial syndromes.

● **HOW TO USE** *Wu wei zi* is included in many patent remedies. It used with *ren shen* (Korean ginseng) and *mai men dong* (lily turf root) to control sweating and tonify *qi* or with warming herbs including *gan jiang* (dry ginger) and *gui zhi* (cinnamon twigs) to disperse Cold and warm the Lungs in asthma and chills.

OTHER ASTRINGENT HERBS

● *Jin ying zi* (*Rosa laevigata*): Cherokee rosehips are used for Kidney *jing* problems and diarrhea.

● *Wu bei zi* (*Rhus chinensis*): nutgalls are used to combat leakage of Lung *qi* causing Deficient Lung; and from the intestines causing diarrhea.

● *Rou dou kou* (*Myristica fragrans*): nutmeg is used to warm the middle *jiao* and control diarrhea.

● *Sang piao xiao* (*Paratendera sinensis*): praying mantis egg cases are mainly used in Deficient Kidney *yang* syndromes.

● *Chun pi* (*Ailanthus altissima*): ailanthus root is used to clear Heat and Damp causing diarrhea or vaginal discharge.

● *Wu mei* (*Prunus mume*): black plum is used to combat leakage in coughing and diarrhea, and to stop bleeding. It is used topically for corns and warts.

HERBS TO TONIFY *YANG*

Tonic herbs—including those for the Blood and *qi* are used to treat Deficiency syndromes and help to strengthen processes in the body. This can include Exterior conditions, and tonics should always be used with caution in lingering superficial syndromes as they can worsen rather than improve the condition. Herbs to tonify *yang* are most often needed for Deficient Kidney *yang* since the Kidney stores Congenital *qi* which is the basis of the body's *yang*. Symptoms can include exhaustion, cold extremities, "cock-crow diarrhea," wheezing, and excessive urination.

Dong chong xia cao caterpillar fungus

BOTANICAL NAME *Cordyceps sinensis*
TASTE Sweet
CHARACTER Neutral
MERIDIANS Lung, Kidney
ACTIONS Stimulates adrenal glands, antibacterial, sedative, hypnotic, some anticancer activity

Dong chong xia cao is a fungus that grows on the noses of certain types of caterpillars. Modern supplies are grown on grain so the caterpillar is no longer essential. The fungus replenishes Lung and Kidney *yang* and also nourishes *yin* making it a balanced remedy for long-term use.

● Avoid if there are external pathogenic symptoms.

● **HOW TO USE** *Dong chong xia cao* is used to boost *yang* energies and *wei qi*. It is used with *xing ren* (bitter apricot) and *chuan bei mu* (fritillary) for Deficient Lung *yin*. Today it is available in powdered form, often mixed with other medicinal fungi, which can be stirred into yogurt or fruit juice.

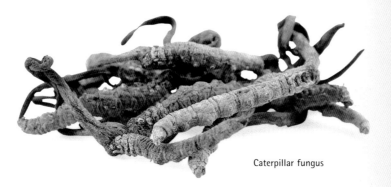

Caterpillar fungus

OTHER SUBSTANCES TO TONIFY YANG

- *Bu gu zhi* (*Psoralea corylifolia*): scuffy pea seed is used to tonify Kidney and Spleen *yang* and treat "cock-crow diarrhea."
- *Hu tao ren* (*Juglans regia*): walnuts are a Kidney *yang* tonic that also nourish the Lung and act as a moist laxative.
- *Ba ji tian* (*Morinda officinalis*): morinda root is used to tonify Kidney *yang* and disperse Wind and Cold-Damp.
- *Yin yang huo*, or *xian ling pi* (*Epimedium grandiflorum*): goatwort is used for Deficient Kidney *yang* and to expel Wind-Cold Dampness.

- *Xian mao* (*Curculigo orchioides*): golden eye-grass rhizome tonifies Kidney *yang* and is used for infertility problems; it also expels Cold and Damp.
- *Hu lu ba* (*Trigonella foenum-graecum*): fenugreek seeds are used for Deficient Kidney *yang* associated with Cold and *qi* Stagnation.
- *Tu si zi* (*Cuscuta chinensis*): dodder seeds are used to tonify the Kidneys in Deficient Kidney *yang* syndromes and also calm the fetus in threatened miscarriage.
- *Du zhong* (*Eucommia ulmoides*): eucommia bark is used for Liver and Kidney *yang* Deficiency and to encourage the smooth flow of *qi* and Blood.

HERBS TO TONIFY *YIN*

These herbs tonify *yin* of Lung, Stomach, Kidney, or Liver and are generally nourishing and moistening. They are combined with other herbs for conditions involving Dryness, Phlegm, or a lack of Body Fluids where symptoms include constipation, dry mouth, thirst, and feverish conditions.

Han lian cao false daisy

BOTANICAL NAME *Eclipta prostrata*
TASTE Sweet, sour
CHARACTER Cold
MERIDIANS Liver, Kidney
ACTIONS Antibacterial, hemostatic

Han lian cao is generally used for conditions that involve tinnitus, premature graying of head hair, teeth problems, and bleeding. In Chinese folk tradition it is used for skin problems such as athlete's foot and dermatitis.

● Avoid in Cold and Deficiency syndromes of Spleen and Kidney.

● **HOW TO USE** *Han lian cao* is combined with *nu zhen zi* (glossy privet berries) for dizziness and premature graying of the hair associated with Kidney Deficiency; with various herbs for different sorts of bleeding, with *ai ye* (mugwort), for example, it is used for uterine bleeding associated with Deficient *yin* syndromes.

False daisy

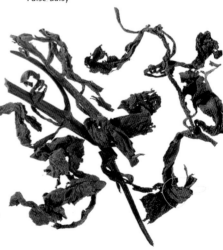

Nu zhen zi glossy privet berries

BOTANICAL NAME *Ligustrum lucidum*
TASTE Sweet, bitter
CHARACTER Neutral
MERIDIANS Liver, Kidney
ACTIONS Antibacterial, cardiotonic, diuretic, immune stimulant

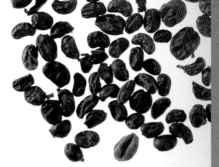

Privet berries

Nu zhen zi nourishes and tonifies the vital essence of Liver and Kidney. Like other Kidney *yin* herbs it helps to restore color to graying hair and also strengthens the knees and waist.
● Avoid in diarrhea with Deficiency of *yang*.
● **HOW TO USE** *Nu zhen zi* is included in various formulae—with *bu gu zhi* (scuffy pea seeds) it is used for dizziness and lower back weakness associated with Deficient Kidney *yin*.

OTHER HERBS TO TONIFY *YIN*

● *Hei zhi ma*, or *hu ma ren* (*Sesamum indicum*): black sesame seeds used to nourish Liver and Kidney *yin*, Blood, and moisten the Intestines in constipation.
● *Mai men dong* (*Ophiopogon japonicus* or *Liriope minor*): lily-turf root is used to moisten the Lung to ease dry coughs and in Heat conditions where *yin* is diminished.
● *Xi yang shen* (*Panax quinquifolius*): American ginseng root used for chronic dry coughs associated with Lung *yin* Deficiency.
● *Shi hu* (*Dendrobium nobile*): orchid stems is good for Deficient Stomach *yin* and to strengthen Kidney *yin*.
● *Yu zhu* (*Polygonatum odoratum*): Solomon's seal root is specific for nourishing Lung and Stomach *yin*, it is used for dizziness associated with Deficient *yin* and Wind.
● *Sang ji sheng* (*Loranthus parasiticus* or *Viscum coloratum*): mulberry mistletoe—both species are used to tonify Liver and Kidney *yin*, expel Wind-Dampness, nourish Blood, and calm the fetus.

SUBSTANCES TO CALM THE SPIRIT

This category includes many non-herbs such as shells and minerals to calm disturbances of Heart *shén* (Spirit) that can lead to irritability, insomnia, and mental disorders. They are divided into two groups: substances to settle the Spirit; and substances that nourish the Heart.

SUBSTANCES TO SETTLE AND CALM THE SPIRIT

Shells and minerals are seen as heavy and solid so weigh upon the Heart and prevent the fluttering of the Spirit which may manifest as palpitations and insomnia. They also weigh down over-exuberant Liver *yang* and redirect Rebellious *qi* downward.

Zhen shu mu mother-of-pearl

ZOOLOGICAL NAME *Pteria margaritifera*
TASTE Sweet, salty
CHARACTER Cold
MERIDIANS Heart, Liver

ACTIONS Little known

As well as settling the spirit, *zhen zhu mu* controls over-exuberant Liver *yang* that can cause eye problems and blurred vision. It is said to help when "Heart and Spirit are not at peace" leading to easy anger, fright, and insomnia.

● Avoid if there is abdominal Cold.

● **HOW TO USE** Mother-of-pearl is used with herbs *dang gui* (Chinese angelica) and *shu di huang* (prepared Chinese foxglove) to calm the Heart and mind and nourish *yin* and Blood. It is used with other minerals and shells for palpitations, anxiety, and seizures or with substances such as *bing pian* (borneol) in topical treatments for sore eyes or ulceration.

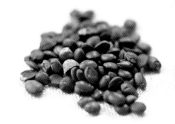

Sour date seed

HERBS THAT NOURISH THE HEART AND CALM THE SPIRIT

These remedies are mainly used for Deficient Heart Blood syndromes causing palpitations and anxiety. Some are also used for Deficient Liver *yin*—they tend to be gentle remedies with few side effects.

Suan zao ren sour date seed

BOTANICAL NAME *Ziziphus jujuba* var. *spinosa*
TASTE Sweet, sour
CHARACTER Neutral
MERIDIANS Heart, Spleen, Liver, Gall Bladder
ACTIONS Sedative, analgesic, hypotensive, lowers body temperature

As well as nourishing the Heart, *suan zao ren* is used to combat abnormal sweating, including night sweats. It is sedating and tranquilizing and eases insomnia, palpitations, and irritability.

● Avoid in cases of pathogenic Fire.
● **HOW TO USE** *Suan zao* ren is combined with *fu ling* (tuckahoe) and *chuan xiong* (Szechuan lovage) in *suan zao ren tang* (sour date decoction) to calm the mind and clear Heat.

OTHER SUBSTANCES THAT NOURISH THE HEART AND CALM THE SPIRIT

● *He huan pi* (*Albizzia julibrissin*): mimosa bark is used for insomnia and irritability but also to invigorate Blood.
● *Yuan zhi* (*Polygala tenuifolia*): Chinese senega root is used to improve the flow of Heart *qi* and clear Phlegm from the Lungs and orifices of the Heart.

FU ZHENG THERAPY

Fu zheng therapy—from *fu*, to strengthen, and *zheng*, constitution—means to restore normality and balance and has been compared with modern Western immunotherapy.

The aim is not to treat a specific disease or infection but to strengthen the body so that innate resistance and energy can overcome the problem. *Fu zheng* can help to increase resistance to disease, prevent tissue damage, destroy abnormal cells, and regulate body functions with allergies, lethargy, repeated infection, and slow wound healing all signs of lowered immunity.

In recent years the *fu zheng* approach has gained in popularity as an alternative therapy for cancer treatments or to combat AIDS. Research into many of the traditional *fu zheng* plants has highlighted their anti-tumor and immuno-stimulating activity. Patent remedies combining *fu zheng* herbs are now readily available. The list of *fu zheng* herbs includes *huang qi* (milk vetch root), *wu wei zi* (schizandra), *nu zhen zi* (glossy privet berries), *gan cao* (liquorice root); *dang shen* (bellflower root), *bai zhu* (white atractylodes), shiitake mushrooms, seaweeds, and Siberian ginseng.

Ling zhi reishi mushroom

BOTANICAL NAME *Ganoderma lucidem*
TASTE Sweet
CHARACTER Slightly warm
MERIDIANS Lung, Heart, Spleen, Liver, Kidney
ACTIONS Antiviral, immune stimulant, expectorant, antitussive, antihistamine, antitumor, reduces blood pressure and cholesterol levels

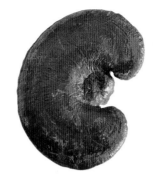

Reishi is the Japanese name for this Oriental bracket fungus that was revered by the ancient Taoists as a longevity tonic. The fungus is used to tonify *qi* and Blood, and also calms the Heart and Spirit. It is traditionally said to encourage determination to live a virtuous life.

● Avoid if there are no signs of weakness or Deficiency.

● **HOW TO USE** *Ling zhi* is taken by itself rather than in combination with other herbs—although extracts are now included in many patent *fu zheng* remedies. It can be eaten like other mushrooms in cooking or made into syrups, tinctures or powders, and is used to stimulate the immune system in both general debility and chronic conditions, including cancer. It is also used for lung problems (including asthma and chronic bronchitis), Heart disharmonies where symptoms include insomnia, palpitations, forgetfulness and hypertension, chronic fatigue syndrome, ME, and AIDS.

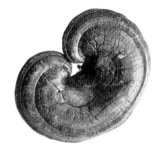

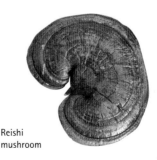

Reishi mushroom

USING HERBAL REMEDIES

Any patient consulting a traditional Chinese medicine practitioner will very likely be sent home with bags of dried herbs to be turned into the daily *tāng* (see also page 132). The mixture will probably be based on a centuries-old formula memorized by Chinese medical students and its choice will have been determined by careful diagnosis.

Increasingly, however, Chinese herbs are found in health food stores, Western pharmacies and on the Internet. Some of these over-the-counter remedies are exact copies of traditional prescriptions, others may be adapted to remove the less acceptable ingredients and others are simply single herbs sold as tinctures or powders.

Very few Chinese herbs are taken as single remedies in traditional therapy—the emphasis is always on combinations and how the remedies work together. Most Chinese herbs sold singly in Western health food shops tend to be tonic remedies and are largely promoted as remedies to

combat fatigue, exhaustion or to stimulate the immune system. These include:

- *Dang gui* (Chinese angelica root): May be marketed as *dong quai*, *dong qwai*, *tang kwai*, or Chinese angelica.
- *Dang shen* (bellflower root): Often sold as codonopsis.
- *Dong chong xia cao* (caterpillar fungus): Also sold as cordyceps.
- *Gou qi zi* (wolfberry fruit): Also sold as lycium fruit or goji berries.
- *He shou wu* (fleeceflower root): Also sold as *fo ti*.
- *Huang qi* (milk vetch root): Often sold as astragalus.
- *Ling zhi* (reishi mushroom): Sold as reishi.

- *San qi* (notoginseng or pseudoginseng root): Sold as *san qi* ginseng or *tian qi*.
- *Shi di huang* (prepared Chinese foxglove root) and *sheng di huang* (fresh or dried Chinese foxglove root): May simply be sold as rehmannia root without any indication of which form has been used. As these two forms of the herb have very different uses care is needed when buying the remedy to be sure the correct one is selected.
- *Ren shen* (Korean ginseng root): May also be sold simply as ginseng, or as Chinese ginseng or red ginseng.
- *Xi yang shen* (American ginseng root): Unlike *ren shen*, a very *yang* herb, American ginseng is cooling, supports *yin* and helps to generate Fluids. It is especially used to nourish Lung *yin*.
- *Wu jia pi* (Siberian ginseng root bark): The whole root is likely to be used in Western products labeled Siberian ginseng rather than simply the bark as is used in Chinese medicine. Siberian ginseng is largely used by Western herbalists as a remedy to combat stress and jet lag.
- *Wu wei zi* (schizandra fruits): Also sold as Schisandra.

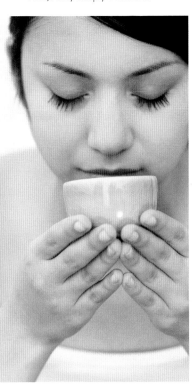

Drinking the traditional *tāng* is often inconvenient for Westerners who prefer pills or tinctures.

USING PATENT REMEDIES

Regulations covering the sale of both single Chinese herbs and patent remedies vary between countries but very few will be licensed by national medicines control agencies and since many are marketed as food supplements, quality can be an issue.

For products made in China, labelling can sometimes be inadequate with plant names given only in Chinese characters or with poorly translated botanical names. Few give details of the traditional cautions associated with the various herbs involved. Packets may suggest dosages but, in accordance with most Western regulations, can give no indication of the therapeutic properties of the product. Equally, it is unlikely that sales staff in many health food stores or pharmacies are trained in traditional Chinese medicine so cannot give informed advice either.

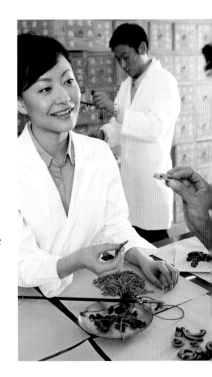

Turning traditional dried herbs into easy-to-take pills or powder has become a common commercial practice.

Some websites selling Chinese herbal formulations strictly control access to qualified practitioners, while others sell to all comers and give minimal information about the products they supply. It is all too easy to buy and take a totally inappropriate remedy. Obtaining an accurate diagnosis and informed advice as to suitable remedies is obviously the safest strategy.

Wherever possible buy from a reputable supplier (products made in Singapore, Japan, or from Western suppliers are often preferable) and check the composition of the formulae against standard lists.

Transliteration of Mandarin Chinese names does vary, with some suppliers using Cantonese rather than Mandarin. Commercializing products can also bring subtle changes in name: a *tāng* (soup) may be made into pills (*wán*) or a traditional powder (*sàn*) also turned into tablets for ease of use and some producers alter the names of formulae to reflect this.

DIGESTIVE REMEDIES

BAO HE WAN

Also sold as "pills for indigestion" or "citrus and crataegus formula," *bao he wan* is used for indigestion, diarrhea, abdominal pains, and gastric flu associated with Food Stagnation. It should not be used if there is gastric or abdominal distention due to Deficiency syndromes. Recommended dosage is generally one tablet or capsule two–three times daily.

Traditionally this contains:
Shan zha (hawthorn berries) **20%**
Shen qu (medicated leaves) **13%**
Lai fu zi (raphanus seed) **20%**
Ban xia (pinellia) **13%**
Chen pi (tangerine peel) **8%**
Fu ling (tuckahoe) **13%**
Lian qiao (forsythia berries) **13%**

HUO XIANG ZHENG QI SAN

"Powder for dispelling turbidity with agastache" is used in acute gastritis and diarrhea associated with Damp-turbidity in Spleen and Stomach and Damp associated with pathogenic

Wind-Cold. It should be avoided where diarrhea is associated with Damp-Heat syndromes. Typical dosage where traditional Chinese pills are used is eight pills three times daily; other products may use larger capsules or tablets.

Traditionally this contains:
Huo xiang (giant hyssop or patchouli) **14%**
Hou po (magnolia bark) **9%**
Chen pi (tangerine peel) **9%**
Zi su ye (perilla leaf) **5%**
Bai zhi (dahurian angelica) **5%**
Ban xia (pinellia) **9%**
Da fu pi (betel husk) **5%**
Bai zhu (white atractylodes) **9%**
Fu ling (tuckahoe) **5%**
Jie geng (balloon flower root) **9%**
Gan cao (liquorice)**12%**
Sheng jiang (fresh ginger root) **6%**
Da zao (black dates) **3%**

RUN CHANG WAN

"Emollient pills" also sold as *ma ren run chang wan* or "moisten intestine pills." Generally used where constipation is due to Blood Deficiency leading to weakness such as following childbirth, or where the cause is Wind leading to Blood Deficiency or Wind-Heat drying the Stomach and Intestines. The mixture should be avoided in pregnancy. Dosage is 3–5 g (usually eight tiny Chinese pills) three times daily. Commercial variants sometimes use flax seed, a traditional Western remedy for constipation, instead of hemp seed and are sold as "linum and rhubarb combination." Two traditional formulae with this name are known.

One contains:
Dang gui (Chinese angelica) **12.5%**
Huo ma ren (hemp seed) **21%**
Sheng di huang (fresh Chinese foxglove root) **42%**
Tao ren (peach seed) and/or **Zing ren** (bitter apricot seed) **12.5%**
Zhi ke (bitter orange fruit) **12%**

While the other contains:
Huo ma ren (hemp seed) **33%**
Dang gui (Chinese angelica) **14%**
Tao ren (peach seed) **26%**
Qing huo (notopterygii root) **13.5%**
Da huang (Chinese rhubarb root) **13.5%**

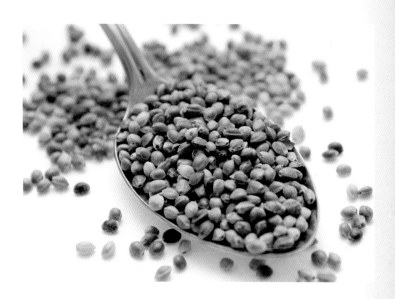

Hemp seeds are traditionally used for treating constipation in the elderly.

SI SHEN WAN

"Pills of the four miraculous drugs" is used for "cock-crow diarrhea" that habitually occurs before dawn due to Spleen and Kidney *yang* Deficiency and Coldness. It occurs at daybreak because that is when *yin* is strongest, and if *yang* is weak then it will not rise and *yin* suddenly descends causing diarrhea.

The remedy should not be used if diarrhea is due to Stagnation or Heat. Typical dosage is up to 12 g of the mixture in pill form taken at bedtime.

Traditionally this contains:
Bu gu zhi (scuffy pea seed) **23%**
Rou dou kou (nutmeg) **12%**
Wu zhu yu (evodia) **6%**
Wu wei zi (schizandra berries) **12%**
Sheng jiang (fresh ginger) **33%**
Da zao (black dates) **14%**

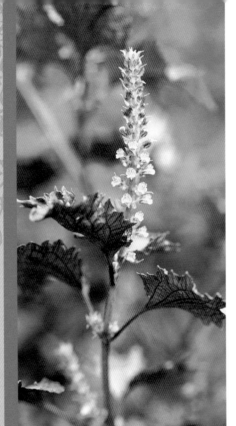

Leaves from the perilla plant are a warming remedy used to treat Cold conditions.

Wind and Cold causing Dryness and interfering with Lung function to cause coughing with thin watery phlegm that may develop into bronchitis. Typical dose is 3–5 g of the powder in water three times daily or the equivalent in tablets.

Traditionally this contains:
Xing ren (bitter apricot seed) **10%**
Zi su ye (perilla leaf) **10%**
Zhi ke (bitter orange) **10%**
Jie geng (balloon flower) **10%**
Qian hu (peucedanum) **10%**
Chen pi (tangerine peel) **10%**
Ban xia (pinellia) **10%**
Fu ling (tuckahoe) **10%**
Sheng jiang (fresh ginger) **10%**
Gan cao (liquorice) **6%**
Da zao (black dates) **4%**

LUNG REMEDIES

XING SU SAN

"Powder of apricot seed and perilla" is also sold as "apricot kernel and perilla formula" in tablet form. This remedy is a diaphoretic to dispel

SANG JU YIN

"Decoction of mulberry leaf and chrysanthemum" is also marketed as "morus leaf and chrysanthemum combination" or "clear Wind-Heat tea pills." Traditionally a decoction, *sang ju yin* is also available in tablet form. It is used to calm coughs and move Lung *qi* in the early stages of warm feverish conditions caused by External Wind and Heat leading to common cold, acute bronchitis, influenza, or conjunctivitis. Avoid where the common cold is due to Wind-Cold or if there is an Internal Heat problem.

Traditionally this contains:
Sang ye (mulberry leaf) **20%**
Ju hua (chrysanthemum flowers) **8%**
Xing ren (bitter apricot seeds) **16%**
Jie geng (balloon flower) **16%**
Bo he (field mint) **6%**
Lian qiao (forsythia flowers) **12%**
Lu gen (reed rhizome) **16%**
Gan cao (liquorice) **6%**

ER CHEN TANG

"Decoction of two old drugs" is also sold as "two-cured decoction" or "citrus and pinellia combination" in tablets and capsules. It is used for Damp Phlegm problems associated with *qi* Deficiency where the Spleen is failing to transport Fluids. Symptoms can include profuse watery sputum, nausea and dizziness. *Er chen tang* is used for chronic bronchitis, emphysema, and coughs.

Traditionally this contains:
Ban xia (pinellia) **30%**
Chen pi (tangerine peel) **20%**
Fu ling (tuckahoe) **30%**
Gan cao (liquorice) **20%**

BU FEI TANG

"Tonify the Lung decoction" is also sold as "ginseng and aster decoction" in tablets and powders. It is used for Lung *qi* Deficiency where there is cough, asthma, or shortness of breath; typically the pulse is feeble and weak and the tongue is pale with a white coating.

Traditionally this contains:
Ren shen (Korean ginseng) **11%**
Huang qi (milk vetch root) **20%**
Sang bai pi (mulberry root bark) **17%**
Zi wan (aster) **11%**
Wu wei zi (schizandra berries) **11%**
Shu di huang (prepared Chinese foxglove) **25%**

LIVER REMEDIES

LONG DAN XIE GAN TANG

"Decoction to purge the Liver Fire with gentiana" is also sold as "gentiana combination" or in pill form as *long dan xie gan wan*. It is used to purge Heat and Fire from the Liver and Gall Bladder as well as clear Heat and Dampness from the *san jiao*. It is used for such conditions as gall bladder inflammation, hepatitis, cystitis, urethritis, prostatitis, and pelvic inflammatory disease as well as associated Liver problems such as conjunctivitis and quick temper. Avoid in Spleen or Stomach Deficiency. Typical dosage is up to seven pills three times daily.

Traditionally this contains
Long dan cao (gentian root) **7%**
Huang qin (baikal skullcap) **14%**
Zhi zi (gardenia fruits) **10%**
Chai hu (thorowax root) **10%**
Mu tong (akebia stems) **10%**
Che qian zi (plantain seeds) **10%**

Gentian root is mainly used to clear Heat and Damp and calm Liver Fire.

Ze xie (water plantain) **10%**
Sheng di huang (fresh Chinese foxglove) **14%**
Dang gui (Chinese angelica root) **10%**
Gan cao (liquorice) **5%**

QI JU DI HUANG WAN

"Pills of six herbs with Chinese foxglove" is also sold as "lycium,

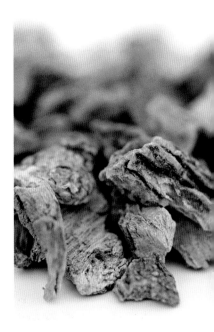

chrysanthemum & rehmannia formula" or "lycii chrysanthemum tea pills." It is used to replenish the vital essence of the Kidney and to nourish the Liver where Liver *yin* Deficiency is the underlying problem. Typical symptoms can include dry eyes and blurred vision with high blood pressure, dizziness, and headaches. Typical dosage is up to 10 g of pills three times daily.

Traditionally this contains:
Gou qi zi (wolfberry fruits) **10%**
Ju hua (chrysanthemum flowers) **7%**
Shu di huang (prepared Chinese foxglove) **17%**
Shan zhu yu (dogwood fruits) **14%**
Shan yao (Chinese yam) **14%**
Ze xie (water plantain) **14%**
Mu dan pi (tree peony bark) **10%**
Fu ling (tuckahoe) **14%**

SI NI SAN

"Frigid extremities powder" is also sold as "bupleurum and *chih shih* decoction," "bupleurum and aurantium formula," "bupleurum and zhi shi formula," or "four pillars tea pills." It is available as an over-the-counter remedy for Internal Heat constraining *yang qi* leading to Stagnant Liver *qi* and Spleen disorders. Typical symptoms include cold fingers and toes, abdominal pain, diarrhea, and liver or gallbladder disorders. The tongue is pale purple with a thin white coating and the pulse is wiry and taut. Typical dosage is eight tiny pills three times daily or up to 9 g in powdered form three times daily.

Traditionally this contains:
Chai hu (thorowax root) **33%**
Zhi shi (immature bitter orange) **22%**
Bai shao yao (white peony) **33%**
Zhi gan cao (prepared liquorice) **11%**

HEART REMEDIES

AN SHEN BU XIN WAN

"Calming the mind and tonifying the Heart pill" is also sold as "Spirit quieting, Heart supplementing pill" and "calm shén, tonify Heart pill." Some products also contain *sheng di huang* (fresh Chinese foxglove). This formula is used to move and nourish Blood where the underlying problem is Deficient Heart Blood with Liver and Heart *yin* deficiency. Typical symptoms include palpitations, disturbing dreams, insomnia, and a tendency for atherosclerosis. Typical dose is two pills, three times daily.

Traditionally this contains:
Zhen zhu mu (mother of pearl) **48%**
He shou wu (fleeceflower) **11%**
Nu zhen zi (glossy privet) **9%**
Han lian cao (false daisy) **6.5%**
Dan shen (Chinese sage root) **6.5%**
He huan pi (mimosa bark) **6.5%**
Tu si zi (dodder seeds) **6.5%**
Wu wei zi (schizandra fruits) **3%**
Shi chang pu (sweetflag rhizome) **3%**

GUI PI TANG

Gui pi tang "decoction to strengthen the Heart and the Spleen" also sold as "ginseng and longan combination," *gui pi wan*, *gui pi pian*, or "restore the Spleen decoction." *Gui pi tang* nourishes the Heart and tonifies the Spleen as well as replenishing *qi* and Blood. It is used for Heart and Spleen Deficiency which can cause insomnia, anemia, palpitations, forgetfulness, disturbing dreams, or menstrual irregularities. It is also said to "calm the mind." Typical dosage is up to eight pills three times daily.

Traditionally this contains:
Ren shen (Korean ginseng) **8%**
Huang qi (milk vetch root) **12%**
Bai zhu (white atractylodes) **11%**
Gan cao (liquorice) **5%**
Dang gui (Chinese angelica) **11%**
Yuan zhi (Chinese senega root) **8%**
Fu ling (tuckahoe) **11%**
Suan zao ren (sour date seeds) **12%**
Long yan rou (longan) **11%**
Mu xiang (costus root) **6%**
Sheng jiang (fresh ginger) **2%**
Da zao (black dates) **3%**

GUA LOU XIE BAI BAN XIA TANG

"Snakegourd, chive, and pinellia decoction" is also sold as "trichosanthes, bakerie, and pinellia combination" used for chest pains and severe coughs. Traditionally wine is added to the final decoction but in over the counter remedies it is generally omitted. *Gua lou xie bai bai jiu tang* is the prescription without the *ban xia* (pinellia) and is used for conditions such as angina pectoris related to Phlegm in the Heart obstructing the *qi* flow and causing Stagnation and *yang* Deficiency. *Ban xia* (pinellia) is added if the symptoms are more severe but always seems to be included in patent formulae. Some products are powders to mix with wine, others are capsules. Dosage varies with the pack.

Traditionally this contains
Gua lou zi (snakegourd fruit) **38%**
Xie bai (Chinese chives) **24%**
Ban xia (pinellia) **38%**
Bai jiu (white wine)

Chinese or garlic chives invigorate *qi* flow and relieve pain.

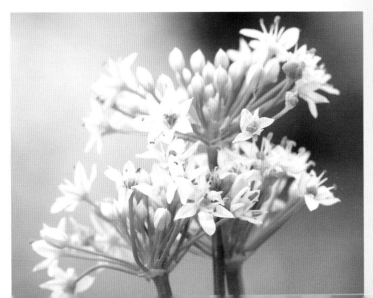

KIDNEY AND URINARY REMEDIES

LIU WEI DI HUANG WAN

"Pills of six ingredients with rehmannia" is also sold as "rehmannia six formula," "six flavor rehmannia teapills," or "six flavor tea formula." It is one of the most highly regarded traditional Chinese formulae; used to nourish Kidney and Liver *yin* and is used for ailments ranging from chronic nephritis to menopausal disorders, urinary tract infections, dizziness, tinnitus, lumbago, deafness, and diabetes. Avoid in cases of *yang* or Spleen Deficiency (where symptoms include indigestion and diarrhea) or where there is Dampness. Typical dose is up to 8 pills three times daily.

Traditionally this contains:
Shu di huang (prepared Chinese foxglove) **28%**
Shan zhu yu (dogwood fruits) **17%**
Shan yao (Chinese yam) **17%**
Ze xie (water plantain) **14%**
Mu dan pi (tree peony bark) **10%**
Fu ling (tuckahoe) **14%**

JIN GUI SHEN QI WAN

"Pills for restoring the vital energy and function of the Kidney" is also sold as "Golden Book teapills," *ba wei di huang wan*, "Kidney formula from the Golden Cabinet," or "Golden Chest Kidney pills." It is used to replenish *yang* or vital function of the Kidney and to warm the lower parts of the body.

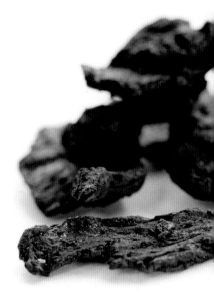

Cooked Chinese foxglove root is used for various menstrual disorders to nourish Blood.

The remedy is used to replenish Kidney *yang* and to warm the lower parts of the body. Symptoms of Kidney *yang* Deficiency include lumbago, coldness in the lower body, pain in the lower abdomen, frequent urination, and persistent diarrhea. Avoid in *yin* Deficiency and Heat syndromes. Typical dosage is up to 8 pills three times daily.

Traditionally this contains:
Shu di huang (prepared Chinese foxglove) **24%**
Shan zhu yu (dogwood fruits) **15%**
Shan yao (Chinese yam) **11%**
Fu zi (prepared aconite) **11%**
Rou gui (cinnamon bark) **6%**
Ze xie (water plantain) **11%**
Mu dan pi (tree peony bark) **11%**
Fu ling (tuckahoe) **11%**

BA ZHENG SAN

"Powder of eight ingredients to correct urinary disturbance" is also sold as "dianthus formula," "eight righteous teapills," or "eight herb powder for rectification." It is sold in pill form as *ban zheng san wan*. This contains *mu tong* (see page 151) so it is important to ensure that suppliers are using *Akebia* spp. It is used to clear Heat and Dampness in the urinary tract, which may be causing frequent or painful urination as in urinary tract infections, cystitis, urethritis, prostatitis, or urinary stones. Avoid in pregnancy and chronic disease with weakness. Typical dose is 1 g of powder per cup of water up to three times daily or up to 8 pills three times daily.

Traditionally this contains:
Mu tong (akebia stems) **11%**
Qu mai (dianthus) **11%**
Bian xu (knotgrass) **11%**
Hua shi (talc) **19%**
Che qian zi (plantain seed) **11%**
Zhi zi (gardenia flowers) **7.5%**
Da huang (Chinese rhubarb) **11%**
Gan cao (liquorice) **7.5%**
Deng xin cao (rush pith) **11%**

JOINT AND MUSCLE REMEDIES

DU HUO JI SHENG TANG

"Decoction of pubescent angelica and loranthus" is also sold in pill form as "solitary hermit teapills" or "tuhuo and vaeicum combination." It is used to dispel Cold and Dampness, replenish *qi* and Blood and tonify Liver and Kidney. Its main use is for chronic arthritis associated with Cold, Wind and Damp as well as sciatica, rheumatism, lower back pain, and weak knees. Avoid in acute stages of rheumatoid arthritis or where there are other Heat signs. Typical dosage is up to 8 pills three times daily.

Traditionally this contains:
Du huo (pubescent angelica) **10%**
Xi xin (wild ginger) **3%**
Fang feng (siler) **6%**
Qin jiao (large leaf gentian) **6%**
Sang ji sheng (mulberry mistletoe) **9%**

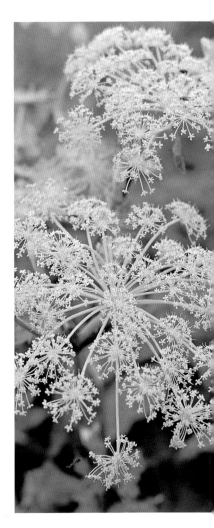

Several types of angelica are used in Chinese medicine—pubescent angelica clears Wind and Damp.

Du zhong (Eucommia) **6%**
Huai niu xi (ox knee root) **6%**
Rou gui (cinnamon bark) **3%**
Dang gui (Chinese angelica) **6%**
Chuan xiong (Szechuan lovage) **6%**
Shu di huang (prepared Chinese foxglove) **9%**
Bai shao yao (white peony) **6%**
Ren shen (Korean ginseng) **6%**
Fu ling (tuckahoe) **12%**
Gan cao (liquorice) **6%**

GUI ZHI SHAO YAO ZHI MU TANG

"Decoction of cinnamon twig, peony and anemarrhena" is also sold in pill form as "cinnamon and anemarrhena combination." It is used to clear Wind and Dampness and to unblock the Channels, eliminate Heat, and relieve pain. It is used for recurrent Wind-Cold-Damp obstructions that can cause localized Heat—such as acute gout, arthritis, joint pain, rheumatism, and joint swellings typified by hot, swollen joints. Typical dosage is up to 8 pills a day.

Traditionally this contains:
Gui zhi (cinnamon twigs) **12%**
Bai shao yao (white peony) **12%**
Zhi mu (anemarrhena rhizome) **12%**
Ma huang (ephedra) **12%**
Fu zi (prepared aconite) **12%**
Fang feng (siler) **12%**
Bai zhu (white atractylodes) **12%**
Gan cao (liquorice) **8%**
Sheng jiang (fresh ginger) **8%**

ER MIAO SAN

"Powder of two effective ingredients" is also sold as "two marvel powder." It is used to clear Heat and Damp leading to low back pain, weakness and pain in the lower limbs, joint swellings especially knees and feet, rheumatoid arthritis, and gout. Avoid where there is Liver or Kidney Deficiency or Lung-Heat. Typical dosage is up to 6 g of the powder taken with ginger juice and warm water three times daily.

Traditionally this contains:
Huang bai (cork tree bark) **45%** .
Cang zhu (gray atractylodes) **55%**

GYNECOLOGICAL REMEDIES

Goatwort leaves help to restore the Kidney so are often used in menopausal remedies.

XIAO YAO SAN

"The ease powder" is also sold as "free and easy wanderer powder," "rambling powder," "bupleurum and *tangkuei* powder," "bupleurum and *dang gui* formula," and "*tangkuei* and bupleurum formula." It is widely used for menstrual and gynecological problems including irregular periods, period pain, excessively heavy periods, and fibrocystic breast problems, It harmonizes Liver and Spleen and also relieves Constrained Liver *qi* and replenishes Blood. Typical dose is up to 4 g of the powder taken in warm water three times daily.

Traditionally this contains:
Chai hu (thorowax root) **13.5%**
Dang gui (Chinese angelica) **13.5%**
Bai shao yao (white peony) **18.5%**
Bai zhu (white atractylodes) **13.5%**
Fu ling (tuckahoe) **23%**
Gan cao (liquorice) **9%**
Sheng jiang (fresh ginger) **4.5%**
Bo he (field mint) **4.5%**

ER XIAN TANG

"Decoction of curculigo and epimedium" is also known as "two immortals decoction," "curculigo and epimedium combination," and sold in tablet form as *er xian tang wan* or "two immortals teapills." Used for menopausal problems, it replenishes vital essence and vital function (*yin* and *yang*) of the Kidney and purges Kidney Fire. It also helps to regulate the *chong* and *ren* channels. The remedy is also used for high blood pressure and urinary tract infection associated with Kidney dysfunction. Typical dose for patent remedies is 3–4 capsules or eight pills three times daily.

Traditionally this contains:
Xian mao (golden eyegrass) **23%**
Yin yang huo also known as **xian ling pi** (goatwort) **23%**
Ba ji tian (morinda root) **13.5%**
Dang gui (Chinese angelica) **13.5%**
Huang bai (cork tree bark) **13.5%**
Zhi mu (anemarrhena rhizome) **13.5%**

Symptoms include pallor, dizziness, palpitations, breathing problems, and fatigue. It is used for such conditions as anemia and heavy menstrual bleeding. Up to 90 g of the herbs are used to make the traditional daily decoction but in tablet form the usual dosage is eight tiny pills three times daily or as directed on the pack.

Traditionally this contains:
Ren shen (Korean ginseng) **9%**
Shu di huang (prepared Chinese foxglove) **18%**
Bai zhu (white atractylodes) **13%**
Dang gui (Chinese angelica root) **14%**
Bai shao yao (white peony) **9%**
Fu ling (tuckahoe) **13%**
Chuan xiong (Szechuan lovage) **9%**
Gan cao (liquorice) **7%**
Sheng jiang (fresh ginger) **3%**
Da zao (black dates) **5%**

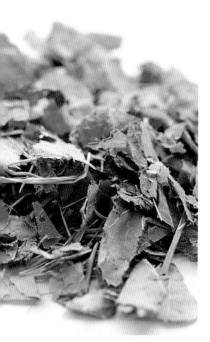

BA ZHEN TANG

"Eight precious ingredients decoction" is sold in pill form as *ba zhen wan*, "eight treasure combination," "*tangkuei* and ginseng eight combination," or "women's precious pills." Used to replenish *qi* and Blood, which is most often associated with blood loss.

SHAO FU ZHU YU TANG

"Decoction for removing Blood Stasis in the lateral abdomen" is also sold as "fennel seed and corydalis combination," "cinnamon and bullrush combination," "*dang gui* and corydalis combination," and "ligusticum and bullrush combination." A popular remedy for period pains, irregular menstruation or uterine bleeding, and lack of menstruation, it invigorates the Blood circulation to clear any stagnation and also warms the channels to relieve pain. It contains flying squirrel droppings and most patent remedies of this combination tactfully just list the zoological name for the animal. Typical dosage of the remedy in tablet form is 3–4 capsules three times daily.

Traditionally this contains:
Dang gui (Chinese angelica) **13.5%**
Pu huang (bullrush pollen) **13.5%**
Chi shao yao (red peony) **13.5%**
Wu ling zhi (flying squirrel faeces) **8.5%**
Mo yao (myrrh) **8.5%**
Rou gui (cinnamon bark) **8.5%**
Chuan xiong (Szechuan lovage) **8.5%**
Yan hu suo (corydalis) **8.5%**
Xiao hui xiang (fennel) **8.5%**
Gan jiang (dry ginger) **8.5%**

YU DAI WAN

"Cure discharge pill" is also sold as "heal vaginal discharge pills," "stop discharge pills," and "femex extract." This formula can also contain *shu di huang* (prepared rehmannia), *dang gui* (Chinese angelica) and *chuan xiong* (Szechuan lovage root) and both the *huang bai* (cork tree bark) and *gao liang jiang* (galangal) should be charred before use. The pills are specific where Damp-Heat is causing leucorrhea (vaginal discharge which is generally yellowish and may smell of fish). The tongue is usually red with a yellow coating and the pulse thready and rapid. Typical dosage of over-the-counter pills is generally eight small pills three times a day.

Traditionally this contains:
Chun pi (ailanthus bark) **60%**
Bai shao yao (white peony root) **20%**
Huang bai (cork tree bark) **10%**
Gao liang jiang (galangal) **10%**

Bullrush pollen helps to encourage Blood circulation so eases the pain caused by Stagnation.

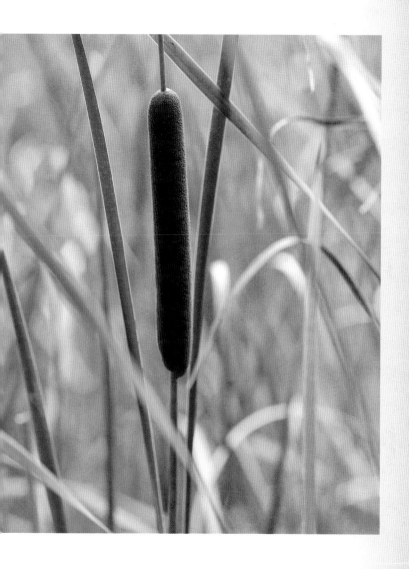

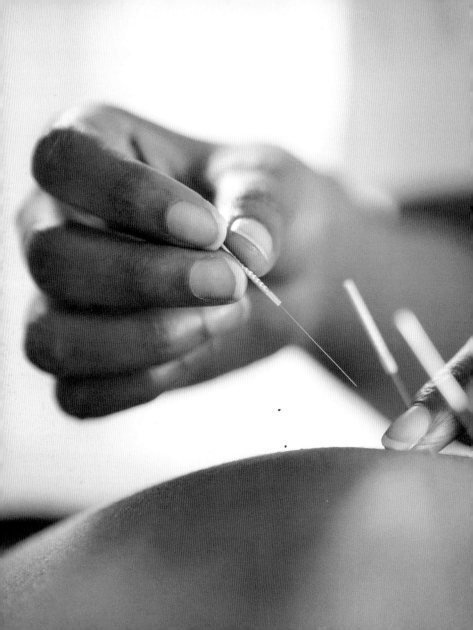

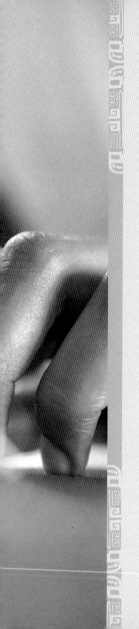

Part 4

ACUPUNCTURE
AND
ACUPRESSURE

THE BIRTH OF NEEDLE TREATMENTS

While Shen Nong is regarded as the father of Chinese herbal medicine, the earliest references to the use of needles in treatment goes back to his contemporary, the Yellow Emperor Huang Di.

The *Yellow Emperor's Classic of Internal Medicine* (see page 10), believed to have been written around 1000 BCE, contains numerous references to the use of needles and acupuncture. Huang Di's physician Qi Bo suggests that acupuncture with flint needles originated from the east while that with the "nine needles" came from the south. Flint needles were used to lance boils or clear pus in infections and also for blood-letting; the finer needles of the south were used in a wide variety of ways. These nine needles each had a specific use:

- arrow-headed (*chan*)—used to prick the skin where external pathogens were moving into the body

- blunt (*di*)—used only on the surface of the skin
- round-sharp needle (*yuan-li*)—for deep needling in *bi* syndrome or carbuncles
- sharp-edged (*feng*)—used for blood-letting and draining abscesses
- ensiform (*pi*)—used to pierce the skin and clear pus
- round (*yuan*)—used for shallow massage for *qi* stagnation
- fine (*hao*)—used for obstruction and joint pain and the forerunner of today's modern filiform acupuncture needles
- long (*chang*)—used in persistent *bi* syndrome and obstructions
- large (*da*)—used in joint disorders and later in hot needling for swellings

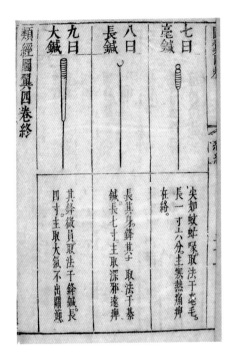

Early Chinese texts detail nine different types of acupuncture needles.

Yellow needles—made from gold, copper, or other yellow metals—were regarded as *yang* and stimulating or concentrating, while white needles—made from silver, chrome, zinc, or other pale metals—were deemed *yin* and calming or dispersing.

Today most modern acupuncturists use fine stainless steel needles ranging from around ½ inch (13 mm) to 5 inches (130 mm) in length and from 0.25 mm to about 0.5 mm in diameter. The thicker needles are generally used for fleshy areas, such as the soles of the feet, and the finer ones for thin skin as on the face or arms.

HEAT TREATMENTS AND RELATED THERAPIES

While acupuncture is perhaps the Chinese therapy best known in the West it is simply one of the "eight limbs" in a total approach to health.

CUPPING

Cupping (*jiaofa*) is a technique that was also once practiced in the West. It involves burning a match inside a small glass sphere to remove some of the oxygen and then placing the cup, open side down, directly onto the skin, which creates a partial vacuum within the cup. This causes the cup to stick to the skin and draw the skin and superficial tissues upward into the cup. The aim is to encourage the flow of *qi* and Blood to the area being treated and clear any local Stagnation, as well as to warm a particular area to expel Cold, Wind, or Damp. Cupping is usually prescribed for dispelling Cold in the Channels, pain, especially joint pain, gastrointestinal disorders, chronic cough, asthma, or paralysis, with the cups placed at appropriate points on the meridians.

The cup may be removed quickly or left in place for ten minutes; the skin underneath becomes reddened due to the congestion of blood flow. Cupping can cause bruising and discomfort if the cup is left in place for too long. Several cups are often used simultaneously.

As well as this sort of stationary cupping, there is also "moving cupping" where the cups are slid across the skin, usually with the help of a little massage oil to make them glide more easily. Sometimes the skin is pricked before the cup is put in place to draw a few drops of blood through the skin. The aim here is to encourage Blood circulation, remove Blood Stasis, or reduce swellings.

MOXIBUSTION

Moxibustion (*jiu*) involves burning dried mugwort (*ai ye*) or "moxa" at relevant points on the meridians.

Cupping is used to treat Cold conditions or relieve pain.

The best-quality moxa is collected by sifting dried mugwort leaves to collect just the fluffy undersides of the leaves, which are then made into cones, cubes, or sticks.

Moxibustion is intended to stimulate circulation of Blood and *qi* and is also used in Cold and Damp conditions—certain forms of arthritis and back pains—to warm and dry an affected area or meridian. In pregnancy, moxibustion treatment is never applied to the lower abdomen.

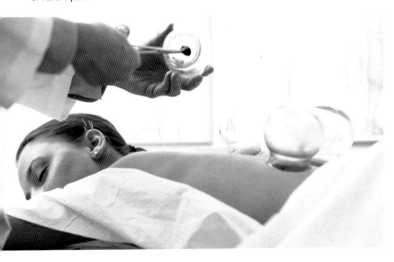

INDIRECT MOXIBUSTION

Moxibustion can be "indirect"—where small balls of moxa are placed on acupuncture needles that are inserted into the body and then lit; or a stick of moxa is lit and held over a particular part of the body. Other substances can also be placed between the moxa and the flesh in the indirect method: moxa may be burned over salt, or on slices of garlic or ginger. Indirect moxibustion can also involve a "moxa box"—boxes of varying sizes that contain loose moxa and cover a large or small part of the body. The moxa is burnt within the box spreading the treatment over a larger area than a single acupuncture needle or moxa stick.

DIRECT MOXIBUSTION

In direct moxibustion, a cone of moxa is placed directly on the body before being lit and generally removed before it actually burns down to the skin. Traditionally it involved blistering and scarring the skin with sore patches that could take time to heal and required regular dressing, however, most

Western practitioners avoid such tissue damage and take care to remove the moxa cone before the skin is reached. Direct moxibustion is never used for the face or head or applied close to important organs, arteries, or bones.

SPOONING

Gua sha is sometimes translated as "spooning" although the term

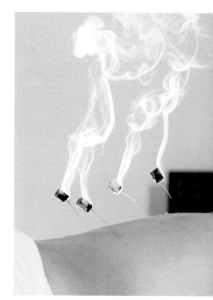

literally means "scrape away fever" and involves repeatedly scraping the skin with a smooth edge—traditionally a ceramic Chinese soup spoon. The skin is oiled and then strokes are made repeatedly along a meridian until the skin is red and appears inflamed. Like cupping, the technique is often used for clearing Blood Stasis and sluggish circulation as well for Lung problems such as asthma, and for painful joints.

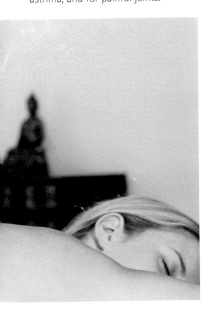

MASSAGE

Tui na is rather like a combination of massage and acupressure that is used to encourage a harmonious flow of *qi* through the Channels and collaterals thus helping the body to heal itself. It combines vigorous massage and manipulation with the use of herbal poultices, compresses and salves. *Tui na* is generally used for pain, joint injuries and muscle sprains.

PLUM BLOSSOM NEEDLE THERAPY

A "plum blossom needle" is made up of a handle, a hammer head and a bundle of needles. Treatment involves tapping specific points or meridians, from gently tapping up to heavier blows which can be painful and may draw a little blood. The technique is used for many conditions—from hair loss to diabetes, obesity, or menstrual disorders.

In indirect moxibustion small pieces of crushed mugwort (moxa) are used to heat acupuncture needles.

MERIDIANS

While the concept of meridians dates back perhaps 4,000 or more years, acupuncture has not always been as highly regarded and widely used as it is today. In traditional Chinese medicine, herbal remedies are seen as the more significant therapeutic approach while even in China acupuncture has been dismissed as irrelevant and ineffective by some.

The earliest extant text, *Zhenjiu Jiayijing (The Classic of Acupuncture and Moxibustion)* by Huangfu Mi (CE 214–282), lists around 349 acupuncture points on the main meridians, and by the 6th century, when China's first medical school, the Imperial Medical College was founded, acupuncture was an established and highly formalized therapy.

However, the arrival of European missionaries and the advent of modern medicine cast the entire concept of acupuncture and meridians in doubt and by 1822 the Imperial College had dropped acupuncture from its curriculum.

China banned the therapy entirely 100 years later. It was only during the 1950s with the revival of interest in traditional Chinese therapies, encouraged by the Communist government, that acupuncture clinics once more appeared along with a renewed scientific approach in the concept.

In the past few decades various scientific studies have demonstrated that acupuncture can be helpful for various types of pain—notably low back pain, headaches, period pain, sprains, and sciatica—as well as relieving conditions including nausea, blood pressure problems, and depression. Acupuncture can

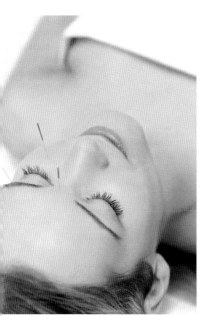

Many practitioners report success with using acupuncture to treat headaches.

also be helpful following surgery to help restore normal *qi* flow and is widely used in traditional treatments for *qi* and Blood stagnation, and disordered *qi* movements.

Medical reports from China also suggest significant success with stroke victims and in paralysis; in many of these cases acupuncture is likely to be only one aspect of treatment, which will probably also include *qigong*, massage, and herbal remedies.

SCEPTICISM

Many orthodox practitioners remain sceptical of acupuncture treatments, with critics describing the meridians as about as real as lines of longitude and latitude. As a therapy it is not always effective even for those conditions where success has been reported and acknowledged by the World Health Organization (WHO).

In recent years it has come in for criticism for hygiene risks (blamed for transmitting hepatitis and HIV although easily overcome by the use of disposable needles), and wrongly inserted needles can also cause bleeding, bruises and, in some people, dizziness. There are rare reports of nerve and kidney damage from needles at certain points, and also miscarriage since some acu-points stimulate production of adrenocorticotropic hormone (ACTH) and oxytocin (both of which stimulate uterine contractions).

In the West acupuncture is regarded as the main form of Chinese medical therapy but in China itself herbal prescriptions for patients typically outnumber acupuncture by around eight to one. Herbs are also almost always given to support the acupuncture treatment. Western acupuncturists are rarely trained in herbal medicine and where they do add herbs to their treatments, they often resort to ready-prepared pills and powders rather than prescribing crude herbs. These patent remedies (discussed in Part 3) can vary in quality, and limited availability also restricts the options available for acupuncturists to use.

Vessel (*du mai*), and the Conception Vessel (*ren mai*). Each of these points has its own Chinese name but they are also referred to using a standard shorthand for the Channel and the number of the point.

Points are also defined in terms of distance from each other or from significant landmarks on the body. These distances are based on the dimensions of the hand. One *cun* is a thumb's width; 1.5 *cun* is two fingers' width and three *cun* is equivalent to four fingers' width. In the West one *cun* is sometimes standardized as 1 inch (2.5 cm) but the size of a *cun* should really be related to the individual involved as obviously a small woman would have a smaller *cun* of 2 cm or less and the relative location of her acu-points would be in proportion.

ACU-POINTS

Today some 361 acu-points are defined on the 12 primary channels and the two most important secondary channels, the Governing

ACU-POINTS		
Name of meridian	Abbreviation	No. of acu-points
Heart (hand *shaoyin*)	HT	9
Small Intestine (hand *taiyang*)	SI	19
Liver (foot *jueyin*)	LV	14
Gall Bladder (foot *shaoyang*)	GB	44
Spleen (foot *taiyin*)	SP	21
Stomach (foot *yangming*)	ST	45
Lung (hand *taiyin*)	LU	11
Large intestine (hand *yangming*)	LI	20
Kidney (foot *shaoyin*)	KD	27
Urinary Bladder (foot *taiyang*)	UB	67
Pericardium (hand *jueyin*)	PC	9
San jiao/Triple Burner (hand *shaoyang*)	SJ	23
Governing Vessel (*du mai*)	GV	28
Conception Vessel (*ren mai*)	CV	24

FINDING THE MAIN MERIDIANS AND ACU-POINTS

Each meridian is replicated on either side of the body so when, for example, the meridian is said to travel down the backbone, one thumb's width from the midpoint of the spine, there are actually two meridians two thumb's widths apart with one on either side of the spine.

HEART MERIDIAN

The Heart meridian starts from **HT1** (*ji quan*) in the center of the armpit, then continues to **HT3** (*shao hai*) just inside the elbow against the bone. **HT5** (*tong li*) can be found one thumb's width above the crease of the wrist when the palm is facing upward. **HT7** (*shen men*) is on the wrist crease in the hollow below the little finger, while **HT9** (*shao chong*) is on the inside edge of the little finger at the bottom corner of the nail.

HEART MERIDIAN

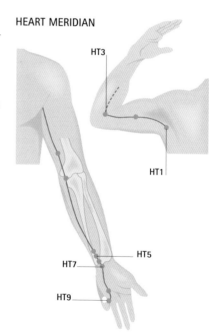

HT3

HT1

HT5

HT7

HT9

SMALL INTESTINE MERIDIAN

SMALL INTESTINE MERIDIAN

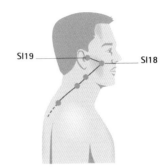

The Small Intestine meridian starts from **SI1** (*shao ze*) on the outside edge of the little finger at the base of the nail, continues to **SI4** (*wan gu*) in the hollow of the hand between hand and arm. **SI5** (*yang gu*) is on the outside edge of the hand between hand and wrist with **SI6** (*yang lao*) in the depression just behind the bony ridge of the wrist bone. The meridian continues along the edge of the arm to **SI8** (*xiao hai*) in the hollow behind the elbow on the outside of the arm. **SI10** (*nao shu*) is directly below the spine of the shoulder blade on its outside edge and the meridian then zig-zags across the shoulder blade and face, via **SI12** (*bing feng*) found in the depression of the shoulder blade when the arm is lifted, to finish to **SI19** (*ting gong*) in the depression formed when the mouth is open between the jaw joint and the central part of the ear.

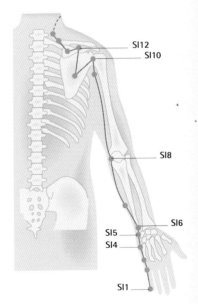

LIVER MERIDIAN

The Liver meridian starts at **LV1** (*da dun*) on the inside edge of the big toe where the nail meets the flesh. **LV2** (*xing jian*) is on the web of skin

LIVER MERIDIAN

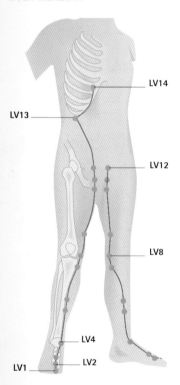

between the big toe and second toe and the meridian then travels up the foot to **LV4** (*zhong feng*) in the depression to the front of the medial malleolus (the protuberance at the lower end of the tibia). From there the meridian moves up the front of the leg to **LV8** (*qu quan*) on the inside of the knee just above where the crease is formed when the knee is bent, to **LV12** (*ji mai*) in the inguinal groove where the femoral artery can be felt, to **LV13** (*zhang men*) at the end of the free 11th rib ending at **LV14** (*qi men*) between the sixth and seventh rib directly below the nipple.

GALL BLADDER MERIDIAN

The Gall Bladder meridian begins at **GB1** (*tong zi liao*) in the hollow at the edge of the eye socket. From there it moves down to the base of the ear and zig-zags up the side of the skull to **GB8** (*shuai gu*) above the top of the ear about one thumb's width inside the hairline. The meridian then tracks back and forth across the skull—down to **GB12** (*wan gu*) in the depression at the base of the bone behind the ear, back across the skull to **GB14** (*yang bai*) on the forehead directly above the pupil about one thumb's width over the mid-point of the eyebrow.

The meridian then travels back via **GB18** (*cheng ling*) on the head about five thumb widths above the hairline behind the level of the ear and above the neck muscles; it then goes down to **GB20** (*feng chi*) at the base of the skull between the muscles, and **GB21** (*jian jing*) a little behind the highest point of the shoulder in line with the seventh cervical vertebra. The line then moves down the body to **GB24** (*ri yue*) directly below the nipple between the seventh and eighth ribs, and **GB25** (*jing men*) on the side of the chest at the free end of the twelfth rib.

The Gall Bladder meridian then moves around the hip joint passing **GB30** (*huan tiao*) between the sacrum at the base of the spine and the protuberance at the top of the femur (thigh bone), and travels down the femur to **GB34** (*yang ling quan*) in the depression at the side of the leg below the knee at the head of the fibula. The channel continues down the leg ending at **GB44** (*zu qiao yin*) one thumb width to the corner of the nail on the outside edge of the fourth toe.

GALL BLADDER MERIDIAN

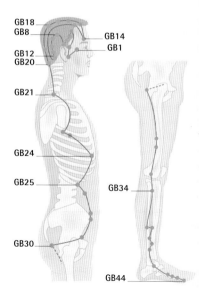

SPLEEN MERIDIAN

The Spleen meridian starts at **SP1** (*yin bai*) at the outside corner of the big toenail and travels along the edge of the foot to **SP4** (*gong sun*) in the depression at the base of the first metatarsal bone. It then moves across the foot and up the leg to **SP6** (*san yin jiao*) four finger widths above the anklebone close to the tibia (shinbone). It continues up the

side of the leg to **SP9** (*yin ling quan*) in the hollow below the knee close to the tibia and **SP10** (*xue hai*) three fingers' width above the knee cap on the bulge of the muscle and is best found with the knee bent.

The meridian continues up the leg to **SP12** (*chong men*) in the groove midway between groin and hipbone, and then up the front of the body to **SP17** (*shi dou*) about a hand's width to the side of the midline of the fifth inter-costal space (between the fifth and sixth ribs). The channel continues upward to **SP20** (*zhou rong*) a little more than a hand's width to the side of the second inter-costal space before making a sharp downturn to end at **SP21** (*da bao*) on the sixth inter-costal space.

SPLEEN MERIDIAN

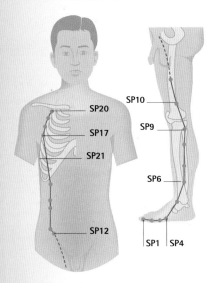

SP20

SP17

SP21

SP12

SP10

SP9

SP6

SP1 SP4

STOMACH MERIDIAN

The Stomach meridian starts at **ST1** (*cheng qi*) below the pupil between the lower eyelid and the eye socket, and moves downward to **ST2** (*si bai*) on the bone of the eye socket below the pupil, and **ST3** (*ju liao*) directly below the eye in a depression under the cheekbone at the level of the wing of the nose. **ST5** (*da ying*) is on the lower jaw in the hollow formed when the jaw muscles are clenched and the cheeks bulged. The meridian then moves upward along the edge of the face to **ST6** (*jia che*) at the

corner of the jaw, one thumb's width toward the nose. **ST7** (*xia gun*) is in the hollow in front of the ear where the upper and lower jaws meet when the muscles are relaxed, and **ST8** (*tou wei*) is on the edge of the forehead above **ST7** half-a thumb's width in front of the hairline.

The meridian then backtracks downward to **ST9** (*ren ying*) level with the Adam's apple to the side where the pulse of the carotid artery is felt, then across to the shoulder blade and down the mid-line of ribs, and across to **ST19** (*bu rong*), two thumbs' width out from the navel and upward to the rib cage. The meridian again continues downward in a straight line to **ST25** (*li mu*), two thumbs' width to the side of the navel and **ST27** (*da ju*) two thumbs' widths below that.

The meridian then moves downward to the leg with **ST35** (*du bi*) found in the depression below the kneecap when the knee is bent. **ST36** (*zu san li*) is three thumbs' widths below **ST35** in the

STOMACH MERIDIAN

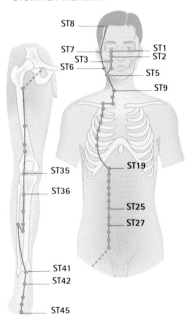

hollow outside the shinbone, and the meridian then moves down the edge of the tibia (shinbone) reaching **ST41** (*jie xi*) on the midpoint of the crease of the ankle when the foot is flexed. **ST42** (*chong yang*) is on the highest point of the foot directly below **ST41** in line with the second and third toes, and the meridian ends at **ST45** (*li dui*) on the outside edge of the second toe in the corner of the nail where it touches the flesh.

LUNG MERIDIAN

The Lung meridian starts at **LU1** (*zhong fu*) in the first inter-costal space between the first and second ribs below the middle of the collarbone and veers slightly upward to **LU2** (*yun men*), six thumb widths to the side of the midline of the shoulder blade, before travelling down the inside of the arm to **LU5** (*chi ze*) on the inside edge of the elbow on the thumb side of the arm. **LU7** (*lie que*) is two fingers' width above the wrist crease, also on the

thumb side of the arm with **LU8** (*jing qu*) below **LU7** in the hollow above the wrist bone. **LU9** (*tai yuan*) is at the wrist crease to the thumb side where the radial pulse can be felt and the meridian ends at **LU11** (*shao shang*) where the bottom of the thumbnail touches the inside edge of the thumb.

LUNG MERIDIAN

LU1

LU2

LU5

LU7

LU9

LU11

LARGE INTESTINE MERIDIAN

The Large Intestine meridian starts at **LI1** (*shang yang*) at the corner of the nail on the index finger on the thumb side of the hand and moves on the outside of the hand to **LI4** (*he gu*) high in the hollow where the thumb and index finger meet. The meridian moves along the edge of the arm to **LI11** (*qu chi*) found at the end of the crease formed by making a 90° angle at the elbow. The meridian continues up the arm to **LI14** (*bi nao*) midway between the elbow and shoulder on the radial side of the arm, and **LI15** (*jian yu*) in the hollow on the outside edge of the shoulder blade. **LI18** (*fu tu*) is level with the Adam's apple in men on the outside edge of the neck and the meridian ends at **LI20** (*ying xiang*) the groove level with midpoint of the wing of the nose.

LARGE INTESTINE MERIDIAN

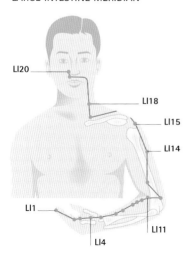

KIDNEY MERIDIAN

The Kidney meridian starts on the sole of the foot at **KD1** (*yong quan*) in the ball of the foot below the second and third toes. It then winds across the foot toward the ankle, first to **KD2** (*ran gu*) in the arch of the foot and **KD3** (*tai xi*) on the inside edge of the ankle between the edge of the anklebone and the Achilles tendon, and **KD6** (*zhao hai*) in the hollow just below the anklebone. The meridian then travels upward to the knee reaching the pubic bone at **KD11** (*heng gu*) then runs parallel to the Conception Vessel (*ren mai*) through **KD14** (*si man*) two thumbs'

KIDNEY MERIDIAN

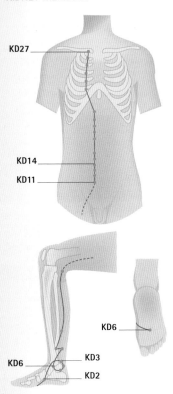

KD27

KD14

KD11

KD6

KD6

KD3

KD2

URINARY BLADDER MERIDIAN

The Urinary Bladder meridian starts at **UB1** (*jing ming*) in the inside corner of the eye. The line then travels over the skull following a line up from the eye, skimming the eyebrow, moving about one thumb's width to the outside of the skull and continuing over the crown to the back of the neck. **UB4** (*qu cha*), **UB5** (*wu chu*), **UB6** (*cheng guan*), and **UB7** (*tong tian*) are all about two fingers' width apart starting with **UB4** just inside the hairline. **UB10** (*tian zhu*) is then below the base of the skull, one thumb's width out from the middle of the neck. The Urinary Bladder meridian then travels down the spine, one thumb's width away from the midpoint of the spine.

UB13 (*fei shu*) is level with the third thoracic vertebra, **UB15** (*xin shu*) level with the fifth thoracic vertebra, **UB17** (*ge shu*) with the seventh; **UB18** (*gan shu*) with the lower border of the ninth; **UB19** (*dan shu*) with the tenth;

width below the navel and slightly to the side. It continues across the rib cage to end at **KD27** (*shu fu*) in a hollow on the lower edge of the shoulder blade.

UB20 (*pi shu*) with the eleventh; UB21 (*wei shu*) with the twelfth; UB22 (*san jiao shu*) with the lower part of the first lumbar vertebra; UB23 (*shen shu*) with the space between the second and third lumbar vertebra; down to UB27 (*xiao chang shu*) level with the first depression in the sacrum. UB28 (*pang guang shu*) is at the third depression of the sacrum in line while UB35 (*hui yang*) is at the tip of the coccyx. The meridian then crosses the buttock to UB36 (*cheng fu*) at the side of the thigh in the midpoint of the gluteal crease and travels down the back of the thigh to the rear before veering upward to UB41 (*fu fen*) just inside the shoulder blade in line with the top of the shoulder.

URINARY BLADDER MERIDIAN

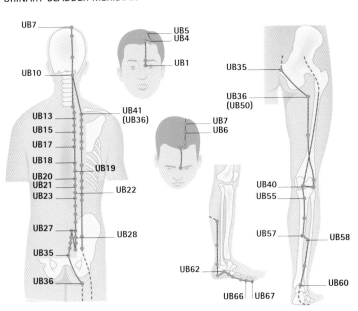

The meridian then runs down the back again, about three thumbs' width outside the spine to rejoin the original path of the meridian at **UB40** (*wei zhong*) at the knee, so that the next point below this is **UB55** (*he yang*) two thumbs' width below **UB40**. The meridian continues down the leg to **UB57** (*cheng san*) two hands' width below **UB40** in the hollow at the center of the calf muscle and **UB58** (*fei yang*) on the edge of the calf muscle, and **UB60** (*kun lun*) on the outside of the ankle between the ankle and Achilles tendon. **UB62** (*shen mai*) is in the depression directly below the ankle bone, and the meridian then moves along the edge of the outside of the foot to **UB66** (*tong gu*) in the hollow at the base of the little toe on the edge of the foot, and ends at **UB67** (*shi yin*) at the base of the little toenail on the outer edge of the foot.

Numbering for this meridian can vary depending on source with some designating **UB41** as **UB36** and then numbering down the spine to designate **UB36** as **UB50**

PERICARDIUM MERIDIAN

The Pericardium meridian starts at **PC1** (*tian chi*) one thumb's width out from the nipple in the fourth inter-costal space. It then moves toward the arm and travels down the inside to **PC3** (*qu ze*) in the crease of the elbow on the inside of the arm, **PC4** (*xi men*) is below it, five thumbs'

PERICARDIUM MERIDIAN

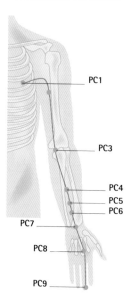

width above the wrist crease and **PC5** (*jian shi*) three thumbs' width above the wrist crease on the inside of the wrist. **PC6** (*nei guan*) is on the inside of the wrist one thumb's width below **PC5** and **PC7** (*da ling*) is in the hollow of the wrist crease below this. **PC8** (*lao gong*) is in the center of the palm where the tip of the middle finger falls when making a loose fist, and the meridian ends at **PC9** (*shong chang*) in the center of the tip of the middle finger.

TRIPLE BURNER MERIDIAN

The *san jiao* or Triple Burner meridian starts at **SJ1** (*guan chong*) on the outside edge of the fourth or ring finger where the nail meets the flesh. It continues across the back of the hand to **SJ4** (*yang chi*) in the hollow at the crease on the back of the hand and **SJ5** (*wai guan*) on the back of the wrist in the hollow where the two bones of the lower arm (the radius and ulna) meet. The meridian then travels up the outside of the arm crossing the elbow and back of the shoulder to **SJ14** (*jian liao*) on the shoulder close to **LI15** and can be felt in a depression when the arm is moved away from the body, and then on to **SJ17** (*yi feng*) at the base of the bone behind the ear to **SJ20** (*jiao sun*) close the ear

TRIPLE BURNER MERIDIAN

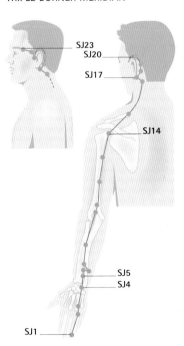

SJ23
SJ20
SJ17
SJ14
SJ5
SJ4
SJ1

but behind it at its highest point. The meridian then follows the line of the ear before crossing the face to end at **SJ23** (*sizhu kong*) in the depression on the outside edge of the eyebrow.

GOVERNING VESSEL

The Governing Vessel essentially runs up the back of the spine from **GV1** (*chang qiang*) midway between the tip of the coccyx and the anus via **GV3** (*yao yang*) on the fourth lumbar vertebra and **GV15** (*ya men*) just below the first cervical vertebra to the base of the skull at **GV16** (*feng fu*). It then crosses the midpoint of the skull and crown of the head reaching **GV20** (*bai hui*) at the top of the skull and moves through **GV23** (*shang xing*) half-a-thumb's width from **GV24** (*shen ting*) at the front hairline and **GV26** (*shui gou*) just below the nose, two-thirds of the way to the upper lip and ends at **GV28** (*yin jiao*) inside the mouth where the gum meets the upper lip.

GOVERNING VESSEL

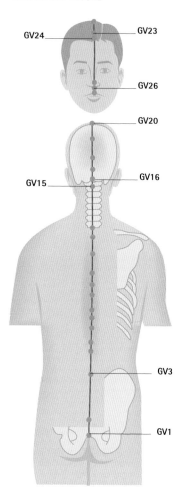

CONCEPTION VESSEL

The Conception Vessel starts at **CV1** (*hui yin*) in the center of the perineum which in men is between the anus and scrotum and in women between the anus and vulva. It then moves up the front of the midline of the body to **CV4** (*guan yuan*) four fingers' width below the navel and **CV6** (*qi hai*) two fingers' width above it. **CV7** (*yin jiao*) is one thumb's width below the navel and **CV8** (*shen que*) in the center of the navel itself. **CV10** (*xia wan*) is then two thumbs' width above the navel and **CV12** (*zong wan*) four thumbs' widths above the navel. **CV14** (*ju que*) is about six thumbs' widths above the navel, **CV15** (*jiu wei*) is one thumb's width above that and **CV17** (*dan zhong*) is in the midline of the breastbone level with the nipples and the fourth inter-costal space. The meridian continues up the breastbone, neck and chin to end at **CV24** (*cheng jian*) in the center of the groove below the lip.

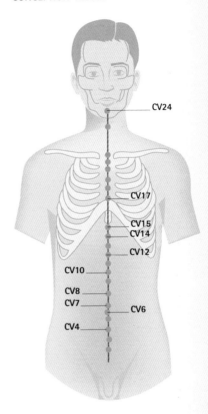

237

SHU POINTS

In Chinese theory there are five specific points on each of the 12 regular channels—known as *shu* or transporting points—that are key in treatment. The points symbolize the movement of *qi* as from a river to the sea and are associated with different stages of a disease and with different groups of disorders.

Jing (well) points are where the "*qi* of the Channel emerges" on the tips of the fingers and toes and are often used to "calm the Spirit" in mental disorders.

Ying (spring) points are where the "qi of the Channel trickles" and are generally close to the *jing* points; they are used to clear Heat in feverish conditions.

Shu (stream) points are where the "*qi* of the Channel begins to pour." They are near to the wrists and ankles and can be used to treat feelings of heaviness in the body as well as pain in the joints such as arthralgia associated with pathogenic Wind and Damp.

Jing (river) points are where the "*qi* of the Channel begins to flow more heavily" and are on the forearm and lower legs; they are used in lung and throat disorders such as coughs and chills.

He (sea) points are where the "*qi* of the Channel links with its related organ" and are near the elbows and knees; they are often used for digestive problems such as diarrhea or to reverse the flow of *qi*.

Each channel also has a "mother point" (*bu xue*) and a "child point" (*xie xue*). The mother point is tonifying and is used in Deficiency syndromes while the child point is sedating and is used in Excess syndromes.

SHU POINTS

Element	Wood	Fire	Earth	Metal	Water
	Jing	*Ying*	*Shu*	*Jing*	*He*
Lung	LU 11	LU 10	LU 9	LU 8	LU 5
Pericardium	PC 9	PC 8	PC 7	PC 5	PC 3
Heart	HT 9	HT 8	HT 7	HT 4	HT 3
Spleen	SP 1	SP 2	SP 3	SP 5	SP 9
Liver	LV 1	LV 2	LV 3	LV 4	LV 8
Kidney	KD 1	KD 2	KD 3	KD 7	KD 10
Large Intestine	LI 1	LI 2	LI 3	LI 5	LI 11
San jiao/Triple Burner	SJ 1	SJ 2	SJ 3	SJ 6	SJ 10
Small Intestine	SI 1	SI 2	SI 3	SI 5	SI 8
Stomach	ST 45	ST 44	ST 43	ST 41	ST 36
Gall Bladder	GB 44	GB 43	GB 41	GB 38	GB 34
Urinary Bladder	UB 67	UB 66	UB 65	UB 60	UB 40

MOTHER AND CHILD POINTS

	Mother	Child
Lung (Metal)	LU 9	LU 5
Large Intestine (Metal)	LI 11	LI 2
Stomach (Earth)	ST 41	ST 45
Spleen (Earth)	SP 2	SP 5
Heart (Fire)	HT 9	HT 7
Small Intestine (Fire)	SI 3	SI 8
Urinary Bladder (Water)	UB 67	UB 65
Kidney (Water)	KD 7	KD 1
Pericardium (Fire)	PC 9	PC 7
San jiao/Triple Burner (Fire)	SJ 3	SJ 10
Gall Bladder (Wood)	GB 43	GB 38
Liver (Wood)	LV 8	LV 2

EAR ACUPUNCTURE

According to the *Nei Jing* (see page 10), the ear "is the place where all the Channels meet;" however, using acupuncture points specifically on the ear has only developed within the past 50 years. The technique was formalized in France in the 1950s by Dr Paul Nogier, although since then it has been accepted in China largely for pain relief.

Some 54 points, mostly on the front of the ear, have been identified and these each correspond to one of the body's organs—some reflect a modern view of anatomy, as with acu-point 27, which signifies the sciatic nerve, others reflect traditional Chinese concepts, such as number 25 usually linked to HT7 (*shenmen* or spirit gate) traditionally used for treating Heart disease.

Ear acupuncture should be avoided in pregnancy and can be inappropriate for the elderly or debilitated; it should be used with caution for those suffering from high blood pressure.

The helix points are used to reduce inflammation, fever and swellings, while ear acupuncturists use the Triple Burner (*san jiao*) point for circulatory, glandular, chest, and abdominal problems. *Shenmen* is used for sedating, as with nervous problems, insomnia, and mental disorders; it is the main point for pain relief, as in arthritis or inflammations; also for dry cough, bronchial asthma, epilepsy, and hypertension.

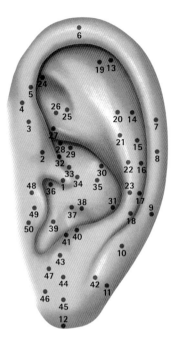

POSTERIOR POINTS (BACK OF THE EAR)

1 upper portion of the back
2 middle portion of the back
3 lower portion of the back
4 groove for lowering blood
  pressure

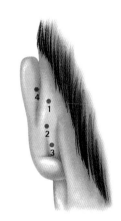

AURICULAR POINTS (FRONT OF THE EAR)

1 diaphragm
2 lower rectum
3 urethra
4 external genitalia
5 sympathetic nervous
  system
6 ear apex
7 helix 1
8 helix 2
9 helix 3
10 helix 4
11 helix 5
12 helix 6

13 finger
14 wrist
15 elbow
16 shoulder
17 shoulder joint
18 clavicle
19 ankle
20 knee
21 abdomen
22 chest
23 cervical
   vertebrae
24 uterus

25 shenmen
26 femoral joint
27 sciatic nerve
28 Urinary Bladder
29 Kidney
30 Liver
31 Spleen
32 Large Intestine
33 appendix
34 Small Intestine
35 Stomach
36 esophagus
37 Heart

38 Lung
39 Triple Burner
40 asthmatic relief
41 testis/ovary
42 internal ear
43 tongue
44 eye
45 tonsil
46 lower teeth
47 upper teeth
48 pharynx
49 adrenal
50 internal nose

VISITING AN ACUPUNCTURIST

While acupuncture is only one therapeutic technique of traditional Chinese medicine (TCM), in the West, healthcare professionals and Western-trained doctors sometimes study acupuncture as a single discipline. Their approach to treatment can often be very different from that of a TCM specialist with the emphasis usually on pain relief rather than redirecting or rebalancing *qi* and Essence.

For the TCM doctor, acupuncture is a small part of the treatment with massage or pointing therapy and extensive use of herbal remedies used as well. Needles are generally inserted lightly into the skin, although they may be pushed deeper in fleshy areas such as the buttock. In some cases a special three-edged needle (*san leng zhen*) may be used to deliberately draw blood.

The needles are usually left for between 20 minutes and an hour. The practitioner will generally move the needle occasionally to stimulate the point. Treatments are generally repeated weekly or twice weekly with a course of treatments running to several weeks or even months.

As well as pain relief in traumatic injury, acupuncture can be helpful for osteoarthritis, although it is generally not suitable for rheumatoid arthritis during the inflammatory stage. Many acupuncturists report that most headaches can be successfully treated and also claim long-term relief for migraine sufferers. Acupuncture tends to be less successful for digestive and respiratory problems. Acupuncture

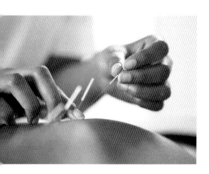

Fine disposable needles may be inserted and left still or moved during treatment.

can be effective in angina pectoris, although as with other chronic conditions, the treatment course needs to be repeated two or three times a year.

The herbs which make up a key component of treatment are generally prescribed on a weekly basis in their crude form to be taken as a *tāng*. Acupuncture obviously needs skill and training and is not a therapy for home use. However, lay people can still make use of its benefits for minor self-limiting problems and first aid by using pressure on the acu-points rather than needles.

CAUTIONS

Acupressure tends to be safe and easy with a few precautions.

- Never apply acupressure to areas of the skin where there are lesions, sores, burns, or scalds.
- Never use acupressure in cases of acute infectious disease.
- Avoid massaging areas where there are lumps or tumors or in the area surrounding the tumor or where the patient may be undergoing radiotherapy.
- Do not use acupressure on patients suffering from chronic heart or liver disease.
- Do not use acupressure on pregnant women unless you are absolutely certain as to the safety of the points pressed as some acu-points can trigger miscarriage.
- Never press so hard as to cause pain or discomfort as that can interrupt the *qi* flow.
- Seek professional help for serious health problems and discontinue self-help treatment if symptoms do not improve within two or three days.

USING ACUPRESSURE

Western "acupressure" derives from the Japanese techniques of *jin shin do*; in China a similar form of acupressure has developed from marital arts and involves manually "pointing" (poking), pressing, pinching, patting, knocking, and pounding acu-points.

Both *jin shin do* and all the Chinese marital arts involve harnessing the *qi* of the body in some way. Pointing therapy makes similar use of *qi* to direct energy to specific points of the body. Pointing therapy is mainly used in China for joint, back and muscle problems and paralysis, while in the West acupressure is often focused on relaxation and stress relief.

One can regard acupressure as a manual pressure on acu-points or as a powerful energy-enhancing technique that involves focusing *qi* into the hands and fingertips and uses the power of vital energy to heal. Preparing to use acupressure involves focused breathing and meditation to help channel *qi* to the hands. Channeling the *qi* to the hands is achieved by a combination of visualization and deep breathing. There are various pressure techniques that can be used and each has its own therapeutic attributes and can be helpful on a wide range of ailments.

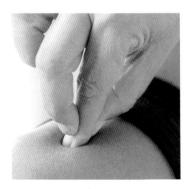

Pointing involves tapping the acu-point quickly with the fingers.

POINTING

There are three hand positions:

1 The index finger is placed on the first joint of the middle finger while the thumb supports the middle finger from below. The ring and little finger are tightly closed.

2 The middle and index fingers are touching and slightly bent, with the thumb under the top joint of the index finger and the ring and little fingers tightly bent.

3 The tips of all five fingers held together with the thumb against the index finger.

In pointing the therapist will knock the acu-point two or three times a second with the hand in one or other of these positions.

PRESSING

This is generally done with the thumb fully extended away from the other fingers with the four fingers made into a fist with the index finger pushing against the second joint of the thumb.

PINCHING

This is only used on nails, toe or finger joints and involves pinching finger or toe between index and middle fingers and scratching the nail or joint with the thumbnail.

PATTING

This involves putting all four fingers together, and slightly flexed, with the thumb against the second joint of the index finger and then patting the meridian gently up to 10 times.

KNOCKING

This has a similar hand position to patting but with the thumb against the first joint of the index finger and knocking with the tips of the fingers rather than the underside.

Modern acupressure techniques are similar to the patting technique, with gentle stroking and the pressing technique using the thumb. Some Japanese-trained therapists prefer the pointing hand-movement but with constant pressure rather than repeated knocking.

DIGESTIVE PROBLEMS

Acupressure can be helpful for easing various abdominal discomforts and digestive symptoms. Note: the position of acu-points is described on pages 224–237.

CONSTIPATION

● **SP12** or **ST25**: These are the usual points to press. Apply gentle pressure for two or three minutes.
● **GB34**: This can be helpful; pressure should be directed toward the inner edge of the fibula. This point is used to release muscular aches and pains as well as constipation and back tension.

INDIGESTION/ FLATULENCE

● **UB21**, **CV8**, and **KD14**: These points should be pressed with a circular motion. UB21 is the main point for stomach-related problems including Food Stagnation and abdominal distention; it is also good

if there is excessive acidity. KD14 is good for flatulence.

DIARRHEA

● **CV6**, **LU5**, and **ST25**: These are all used for diarrhea. ST25 is the main point for all Intestine problems and so can also ease constipation and dysentery. Use the pressing technique with a circular motion.
● **CV4**: is used for "cock-crow diarrhea" associated with Kidney Deficiency.

ACUTE GASTROENTERITIS

● **Yaoyan**: One of the key points that does not sit on any of the main meridians. *Yaoyan* is four and a half fingers' width to the side of the fourth lumbar vertebra (GV3). Pointing and knocking with the fingers should be applied to the point on either side of the spine.

Feizhong and **jingzhong**: These points at the back of the leg, either side of the calf muscle at its widest point, are also used in a similar way.

CV4: Pointing and knocking at CV4 is also used.

NAUSEA / VOMITING

ST36, **PC6**, and **CV12**: The points, commonly used for nausea, should be pressed with a slight circular motion.

CV17, **CV10**, **ST36**, **PC6**, and **SP4**: These points are used for vomiting. Use pointing and knocking for more severe cases or gentle pressure in milder cases. CV17 helps to direct *qi* downward.

GB20: This point is for nervous vomiting associated with Excess Liver *qi* attacking the Stomach. Use pointing and knocking as well as pinching on the roots of the toenails and heel tendon.

TRAVEL SICKNESS

PC6 and **ST36**: PC6 is key point for all forms of nausea including sea sickness, both it and ST36 are easily accessible when traveling and can relieve feelings of nausea.

LV2: Less convenient although equally effective is LV2. In each case press the point firmly for 2–3 minutes with a slight stirring action as you relieve the pressure.

HICCOUGHS

In Chinese medicine hiccoughs are associated with rising Stomach *qi*.

CV15 and **CV14**: These are pressed or pointed and knocked and then gently massaged using the thumb.

SJ17 and **ST36**: Press these points firmly for up to a minute with a slight stirring action as you relieve the pressure.

LUNG AND CATARRHAL PROBLEMS

Note that the position of acu-points is described on pages 224–237. Review these before you begin any treatment.

INFLUENZA AND COMMON COLDS

● **GV16** and **SJ5**: Pressing either of these firmly for 2–3 minutes several times during the day can help to relieve symptoms of influenza.
● **LU7**: This is a useful point to press for common colds.

NASAL CONGESTION AND SINUSITIS

● **LI20**, **ST3**, **GV23**, and **UB10**: For general nasal congestion these can be helpful. Press firmly with the thumb for one or two minutes.
● **GV23** and **UB20**: GV23 is the main point for nose problems including nasal polyps, all forms of

rhinitis and sinus headaches. For sinusitis UB20 is also sometimes used in a similar way—both it and GV23 are well away from the sensitive areas of the face that can become tender in sinus congestion.
● **Yintang**: This point (see headache page 250) is also used for sinus congestion and headache. Use the same pressing technique as above.
● **LU9**: This can be useful if there is a constant watery nasal discharge.

COUGHS

● **LU1**, **LU2**, **LU9**, **CV17**, and **PC3**: These points are used to relieve coughing, with points pressed firmly for 2–3 minutes and a slight stirring action as you relieve the pressure.

ASTHMA

Do not attempt acupressure if someone is having an asthma attack.

● **LU1**, **LU2**, **LV14**, **UB13**, and **CV17**: These point are for general supportive treatment after an attack, using gentle patting techniques. UB13 is also used for other Lung disorders and can be usefully massaged regularly in cases of Lung weakness or recurrent respiratory problems.

● **KD3**: This point is used in asthma due to Kidney Deficiency.

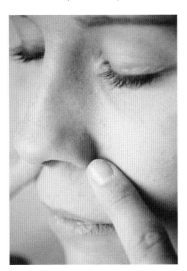

BRONCHITIS

● **LU1**, **LV14**, and **UB13**: Do not apply acupressure in cases of acute bronchitis related to infection but for chronic conditions it can be helpful—use gentle pressing.

LARYNGITIS AND HOARSENESS

● **PC1**: Sometimes used for laryngitis, this can be pressed for up to a minute at regular intervals.

● **LI18**: Used for hoarseness and sudden loss of voice associated with *qi* obstruction in the throat.

SORE THROAT

● **LI2**, **LU5**, **LU10**, **LU11**, and **KD6**: The pointing and knocking technique can be used for up to a minute. LI2 is especially useful if there is gum inflammation or a dry mouth.

Pressing the area around LI20 can help to ease many types of nasal congestion.

ACHES AND PAINS

Note that the position of acu-points is described on pages 224–237. Review these before you begin any treatment.

HEADACHE

● **Yintang**: One of the most popular points for treating headaches, found midway between the inner edges of the eyebrows. It is used to calm the Spirit and to treat insomnia, anxiety and stress a well as sinus problems. Press with thumb or forefinger for several minutes.

● **GV20**, **GB21**, **UB10**, **SI1**, **LI4**, and **LV1**: These points can be similarly pressed for several minutes to relieve headache. GV20 is a main point for headache as well as eye pain and redness associated with Excess *yang* in the upper part of the body. LI4 should not be pressed in pregnancy but is especially good for frontal or sinus pain.

Pressing the areas around GB21 can help to relieve certain headaches.

MIGRAINE

● **UB7**, **GB12**, **GB8**, and **GB20**: These points are most commonly pressed for migraines. In each case press the point firmly for 2–3 minutes with a slight stirring action as you relieve the pressure.

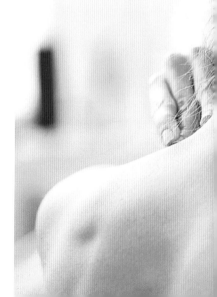

NECK PAIN

● **SI12**, GB20, **GB21**, and **UB7**: These points used for neck pains are readily accessible for self-treatment. Apply gentle pressure for up to two minutes with a slight circular motion as pressure is relieved.

● **UB10**: This is more suitable for neck sprain and stiffness.

● **UB58**: This point is for neck stiffness associated with Wind-Cold. Use the same technique as above.

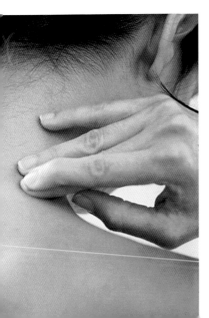

SHOULDER PAIN

● **SI10**, **LI15**, **SJ14**, and **GB21**: Use these points for frozen shoulder applying firm pressure for up to 3 minutes repeated several times daily. GB21 can also be helpful for sprained shoulder joints.

● **SI12**, **LI15**: For more general shoulder pains and stiffness LI15 and SI12 are used with gentle pressure in milder cases and a firmer touch when the pain is severe.

ELBOW PAIN

● **SJ5**, **LI11**, and **LU5**: These points are commonly used for elbow pain while LI11 is more specifically used for sprains. LU5 is good for tendonitis and tennis elbow. The degree of pressure applied should be in proportion to the pain suffered, with greater pressure for more severe pains. Press firmly with the thumb on the point for 2–3 minutes.

WRIST PAIN

● **SJ4**: Wrist pain is best treated by using this point, pressing firmly with the thumb or pointing with the fingers for 2–3 minutes. In pointing therapy the fingernails and finger joints of the affected hand would also be pinched and manipulated two or three times.

LOWER BACK PAIN AND LUMBAGO

● **UB23** and **UB60**: The main points used for chronic low back pain, apply firm pressure on either side of the spine for 2–3 minutes.

● **UB40**: This is sometimes called the "lumbar command" point and can be useful for both lower back pain and problems with the lower limbs.

● **UB58**: This point on the leg can help especially where there is weakness in the lower limbs associated with Kidney Deficiency. Use the same pressing technique as above.

SCIATICA

● **UB36**, **UB57**, and **GB30**: These are all used for sciatica. Apply firm pressure with the thumb on either side of the spine with UB36; to each buttock with GB30 or both legs on UB57. Use firm pressure with the thumbs for 2–3 minutes or pointing and tapping with the fingers for several minutes.

● **Yaoyan**: The extraordinary point, four-and-a-half fingers'-width to the side of the fourth lumbar vertebra (GV3), is also used for sciatica using the heavier pointing technique.

KNEE PAIN

● **ST35**, **SP9**, and **xiyan**: ST35 and SP9 are used for knee pain while the extraordinary point *xiyan* to the side of ST35 in the knee depression below the knee cap, is a specific for all sorts of knee problems including both pain and inflammation. Press firmly with the thumbs for several minutes.

ANKLE PAIN

● **KD3**: One of the main points for treating ankle pain and sprains, this is close to the Achilles tendon. Apply pressure in proportion to the pain (the more pain, the more pressure) or pointing and tapping techniques can be used. In pointing therapy the roots of the toenails and toe joints would also be pinched two or three times.

TOOTHACHE

● **ST6**, **SI18**, and **ST7**: For toothache ST6 is generally used, while SI18 and ST7 are more specific for pain in the upper jaw. Both firm pressure and the pointing and tapping technique can be used.

ST35 and *xiyan* used for knee pain are below the knee cap—level with the demonstrator's forefingers.

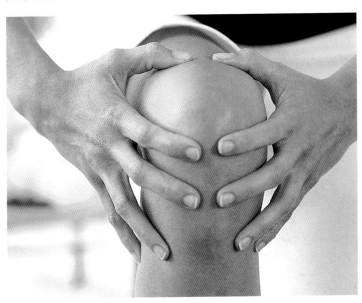

GYNECOLOGICAL AND URINARY PROBLEMS

Note that the position of acu-points is described on pages 224–237. Review these before you begin any treatment.

CYSTITIS AND URINARY PROBLEMS

● **GB25**: This is a diuretic point especially effective for urinary retention or pain and difficulty with passing urine. Press gently or use the gently pointing technique for 1–2 minutes.

● **LV8**, **UB27**, and **UB28**: These are useful points for cystitis and problems with urination. UB27 is especially effective for genito-urinary problems in men including impotence while SP6 can also be helpful.

KIDNEY DISORDERS

● **KD1** and **GB25**: Kidney problems really need professional help but KD1 can be useful to tonify Kidney *yin* and to clear Heat from the Kidney which may be causing thirst and low back pain. GB25 is used for urinary stones and can be helpful for pain relief while awaiting professional treatment. Press firmly for 2–3 minutes with a slight stirring motion as you relieve pressure.

PREMENSTRUAL SYNDROME

● **LU7**, **SP6**, and **SP10**: These points are used for various gynecological problems including premenstrual syndrome. LU7 is the master point of the Conception Vessel and is used often with KD6 to treat both genito-urinary and gynecological problems.

SP6 is used to tonify *yin* and Blood. Press the points gently for 2–3 minutes on a daily basis from mid-cycle until menstruation.

IRREGULAR MENSTRUATION

● **SP10**: This point is used for any gynecological problem associated with Blood, Heat, Stagnation, or Deficiency including irregular menstruation, period pains and premenstrual syndrome.

PERIOD PAIN

● **SP10**, **CV4**, **qipang**, and **yaoyan**: Points used for period pain include SP10, CV4 and *qipang*, which can be found by using the width of the mouth as a measure to create an imaginary equilateral triangle with the navel at the apex: the two lower points are then *qipang*, and *yaoyan* (see sciatica page 252). CV4 and *qipang* should be pressed firmly for 2–3 minutes and then *yaoyan*.

BREASTFEEDING PROBLEMS

● **SI1**: Used for all sorts of breast disorders including insufficient milk and mastitis, this point is at the side of the little fingernail so is ideal for using the pinching technique.
● **PC1**: This can also be pressed for insufficient milk flow.

LABOR

● **UB60** and **UB67**: Useful points to press to ease labour pains are UB60, which can also encourage discharge of the placenta, and UB67, which is sometimes treated with moxa to help turn the baby if a breech birth is likely.

OTHER PROBLEMS

Note that the position of acu-points is described on pages 224–237. Review these before you begin any treatment.

EYE PROBLEMS

● **UB18**: This is one of the most useful points for eye problems—although not one that is easy to reach in self-treatment. Pressing here can be helpful for blurred vision, red or itching eyes, dryness, and eye pain.

● **GB14**: This is mainly used for itching, red eyes.

EAR PROBLEMS

● **SJ17** and **GB12**: The point SJ17 is used for ear problems caused by Wind-Cold including tinnitus, deafness, and earache while GB12 is also used for tinnitus. Press gently for 2—3 minutes or use the pointing technique regularly.

ANXIETY, STRESS, AND EMOTIONAL PROBLEMS

● **HT3** and **HT7**: In Chinese medicine anxiety, poor concentration or memory, depression, and nervousness are often related to disorders of the Spirit. HT3 and HT7 are useful for Phlegm and Heat problems invading the Spirit and causing anxiety, insomnia or manic behavior. HT3 also helps to move *qi* and Blood while HT7 is more tonifying. HT7 is also useful for stress causing palpitations, panic or fear.

● **PC4** and **PC6**: While PC4 is used for Spirit disorders associated with Blood Stasis or *yin* Deficiency, PC6 is useful for Spirit problems associated with both Deficiency and Excess causing mania, nervousness, stress and poor memory. Press firmly for 2—3 minutes or use the pointing technique.

UB15: This is useful for Heart-related emotional disorders causing palpitations, anxiety, stress or poor memory. Use the same technique as above.

FATIGUE

ST36 and CV4: These points are used to help tonify *qi*, Blood, *yin* or *yang* that may be contributing to fatigue and exhaustion. ST36 is used to tonify *qi*, Blood and also the defence energy, while CV4 is useful for Deficiencies. It is an important point for Congenital *qi*, where Deficiency can contribute to feelings of exhaustion, weakness, and chronic fatigue.

CV6: This is a good point for general *qi* tonification. For all points, press firmly for up to 3 minutes.

INSOMNIA

Insomnia in Chinese medicine can be associated with various imbalances from disturbance to the Spirit (*shén*) to Kidney Deficiency or Excessive joy. Obviously identifying the cause is important to choose the appropriate treatment method.

ST45: On the outer edge at the base of the second toe nail, this calming point is especially helpful for insomnia associated with heat or disturbances of the Spirit.

UB15: The main point for insomnia, it is useful for emotional issues related to the Heart, which can be linked to joy, so can be helpful where this is causing insomnia.

SP6: A point used to tonify *yin* and Blood, this is helpful where insomnia is associated with anxiety and emotional upsets.

HT7: This tonifies Heart, *qi*, Blood, *yin* and *yang* and is appropriate for emotional problems causing insomnia and difficulty in concentrating.

PC6: This point is also used for insomnia related to Spirit disorders, both Excess or Deficiency, where other symptoms can include mania, stress, poor memory, and forgetfulness.

DAILY ACUPRESSURE ROUTINES

While acupressure is used in Chinese medicine as a therapeutic technique in ill health, it is also popular in the West for self-massage as an invigorating treatment in the morning and a more relaxing approach at the end of the day.

Typical morning routines start by rubbing the palms vigorously together for about 30 seconds to stimulate the *qi* flow and then tapping all over the scalp with the fingertips as though drumming. Next rub the fingertips downward over the face as though the fingers were a rake (this is not advisable if you have long finger nails) and end by pinching the eyebrows between thumb and forefinger starting at the inner edge of the eyebrow and moving outward on an outward breath. These actions stimulate both digestive and lymphatic systems and can make an invigorating start to the day.

To encourage *qi* flow to the Lungs and Heart place the hands palm down on the cheeks with fingertips pointing upward and then rub the hands up and down as fast possible. Repeat the rubbing action on either side of the nose for at least three out-breaths.

Regular massage of the meridians is also advocated by some acupressure therapists. Stretch out the right arm so that the palm is facing downward and the hand pointing to the floor. Then with the left hand make a fist and gently pound the inner surface of the arm from shoulder to hand starting with the inside edge of the arm then repeating along a center line and finally on the outside edge. This stimulates the Heart, Pericardium, and Lung meridians. Turn the hand over and repeat the process pounding along the back of the arm—again starting with the inner edge, then in the center and finally the outside edge. This stimulates the Small Intestine, *san jiao* and Large Intestine meridians. Finally rotate the arm in a windmill movement in front of the body and shake it vigorously at the wrist. The entire exercise should then be repeated with the left arm, pounding with a loose fist of the right hand.

Relaxing massage is not easy to administer on oneself but UB10 (*tian zhu*) and GV15 (*ya men*) are within easy reach at the back of the neck and both are ideal points for easing neck stiffness that can so often be a cause of tension headaches. Pressing these points for several minutes can often help to ease physical manifestations of stress that build up after a day at work—and the points are easily reached even while sitting on a commuter train on the journey home.

Pinching the eyebrows can be part of an invigorating morning routine.

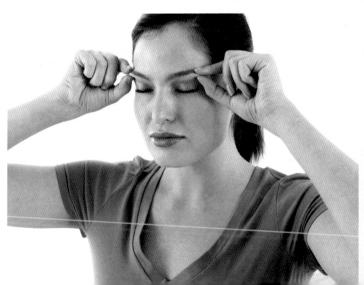

BABY MASSAGE

Acupuncture and acupressure are inappropriate for small children and babies—the meridians are too close together. Instead massage is used gently rubbing a finger or fingers along the meridian to stimulate certain bodily functions or ease discomfort.

Baby massage (*tui na*) is especially suitable for colic, coughs, diarrhea, irritability, and sleeplessness, and is also used to strengthen the *wèi qi* (immune system) and invigorate Blood. Regular massage is also good for the mother, increasing bonding and easing post-natal depression.

HAND AND ARM MASSAGE

Usually just the baby's fingers, arms or legs are massaged rather than a full-body massage common with adults. Treatment needs to be very gentle with none of the vigorous pressing or pushing associated with adult massage techniques, instead repeated stroking is generally used.

For indigestion, vomiting, and poor appetite, for example, the Chinese mother will simply stroke her finger in a rolling circular motion clockwise on the baby's palm—not once or twice but around 200 times. This is the *nèibagua* point, which helps to strengthen Spleen and normalize digestion.

The *pijing* point on the palm side of the first top thumb joint, can be helpful for easing constipation and diarrhea: for diarrhea rub the baby's thumb from tip to base up to 200 times; for constipation stroke from the base of the thumb toward the tip up to 200 times. Alternatively use *xinjing* on the top joint of the middle finger—stroke toward the palm to give relief from diarrhea and away from the palm for constipation. For acute indigestion rub the *banmen* point at the base of the thumb clockwise up to 100 times. *Feijing* at the top joint of the ring finger can be held firmly for 30 seconds or so to ease common colds, coughs, and constipation.

The *zongjin* point at the mid-point of the wrist crease on the palm is a good point to soothe convulsions, mental stress, diarrhea, vomiting, and ulcer: massage the point pressing gently up to 20 times. The

yujijiao point just above the *zongjin* point moving toward the palm is also useful for calming the baby, easing sore eyes and soothing excessive crying—it should be tapped lightly with a pointing finger 7–8 times to clear pathogenic Heat, and ease red, sore eyes, and excessive crying.

The *neilaogong* point in the center of the palm is used for reducing the fevers of common colds and excess heat as well as easing problems caused by fright: the palm should be

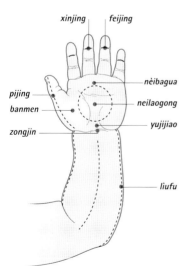

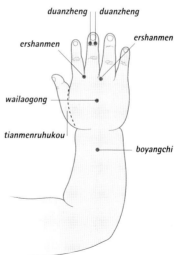

rubbed gently with a clockwise motion up to 100 times. On the inner side of the forearm is the *liufu* point used to cool the baby during heat spells if the infant is suffering from Heat problems—gently stroking the inner side of the arm with a circular motion can help.

Gently stroking on the back of the hand from the middle of the forearm toward the wrist up to 100 times (the *boyangchi* point) can help the circulation and provide relief from digestive upsets while pressing the tips of all five fingers three times can be good to relieve crying fits.

The *wailaogong* point in the center of the back of the hand can be massaged gently for up to five minutes to ease diarrhea and excessive tummy rumblings. *Tianmenruhukou*, between the thumb and the index finger on the back of the hand, can be pressed up to 100 times to ease sore throats, clenched teeth and chest problems, while *ershanmen*, the center of the top of the hand in the depression between the second and third fingers, can help encourage circulation of Blood and *qi*, and easing common cold symptoms—it should be pressed gently five times. *Duanzheng*, at the base of the nail on the middle finger, is used to ease diarrhea, and vomiting—squeeze the sides of the baby's middle finger between your thumb and index finger up to 25 times.

FACE, LEGS, AND CHEST MASSAGE

Massage on the face, legs and parts of the chest can be used especially in toddlers. Techniques for calming restless infants include placing both thumbs on the baby's forehead just above the eyebrows and stroking alternately with the thumbs from eyebrow to hairline, repeated slowly and gently 100 times or until the baby calms.

Massaging the *tianmen* point—in the center of the forehead at the hairline—by lightly stroking from the

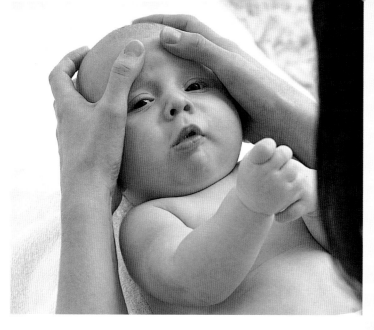

Stroking the forehead from eyebrow to hairline can soothe restless infants.

middle of the forehead to eyebrows to the top of forehead to hair is said to relieve convulsions, spasm, eye tension, blurred vision, dizziness, or nasal congestion.

For coughs and vomiting, gently stroking the middle of the breast bone (*tanzhong* acu-point) with a circular movement 50–100 times can be helpful. For ear problems including infections and earaches stroke gently from the center of the chin across toward the edges of the jaw (*yanguan*) 100 times.

Points on the abdomen—such as *dujiao* just below the navel and *duqi* at the navel—can be massaged gently for digestive upsets, while *rugen*, just below the nipple, can be massaged gently for 30 seconds or more to give relief from productive coughs.

263

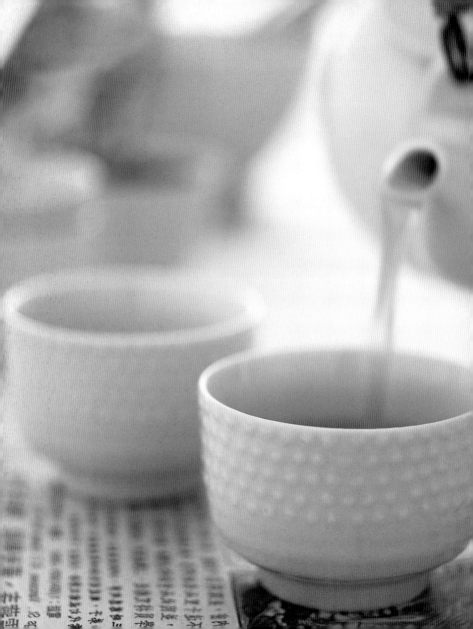

Part 5

UNDERSTANDING
CHINESE FOOD
CURES

CHINESE DIETARY THERAPY

Dietary therapy—*ch'ang ming*—is seen as the third of the "eight limbs" of Chinese medicine. It is closely associated with herbal treatments, with similar underlying theories as to the character and therapeutics of the food we eat.

Rather than considering foods as sources of protein, carbohydrates, vitamins, or calories, Chinese theory sees food in terms of taste, energy and movement. Food is used—much as herbs are—to balance the body's energies and improve general health. There are foods, for example, to strengthen the five *zang* organs, to improve defence energy or the body's immune system, to nourish Blood, jīng or shén, to ensure *yin-yang* balance, to restore health after childbirth or combat the effects of ageing. In addition, many Chinese medicinal herbs are used in cooking to create therapeutic dishes. Certain foods are also eaten at particular times of year as preventatives for seasonal ills caused by external pathogens such as Cold or Damp.

While food can be used to combat the effects of the seasons, the ancient Taoists believed it was important to be at one with the environment, so there is a tradition of eating pungent, hot foods in the summer and bitter, cold foods in the winter in order to retain this vital harmony and *yin-yang* balance. As the great herbalist Li Shi Zhen put it in the 16th century:

"In spring one should eat more pungent and warm foods to stay in harmony with the upward movement of the season; in summer one should eat more pungent and hot foods to stay in harmony with the outward movement of the season; in autumn one should eat more sour and warm foods to stay in

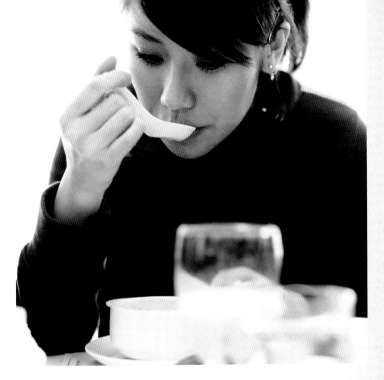

harmony with the downward movement of the season; in winter one should eat more bitter and cold foods to stay in harmony with the inward movement of the season."

As with Chinese medicine, dietary therapy is based on the five-element model and the concepts of *yin* and *yang*. Chinese foods have five flavors and five energies, and they can also

In Chinese theory food is seen in terms of taste, energy and movement.

have different movements within the body and impact different organs. Through the five-element model, taste is linked to specific organs—such as sour food is associated with Wood and the Liver—so a surfeit of any particular taste can cause imbalance in the associated organ.

FIVE TASTES

The five tastes of Chinese foods are pungent (also described as acrid), sweet, sour, bitter and salty. Many foods can have two flavors simultaneously—raspberries and apples, for example, can be both sweet and sour at the same time.

PUNGENT FOODS

These include many culinary herbs, such as parsley, cloves and coriander, several members of the onion family (spring onions, garlic, chives) as well as ginger and kumquats. Pungent foods are described as dispersing and flowing: they can cause sweating, help to clear toxins from the body and also encourage *qi* circulation.

SWEET FOODS

These include honey, sugar, and many fruits, including cherries, bananas, watermelon, and pineapple. Sweet foods tend to be highly nutritious and many grains are also defined as sweet, while several types of meat combine sweetness with other flavors. These foods can neutralize the toxic effects of other foods and also ease acute symptoms.

SOUR FOODS

Also described as astringent, these include lemons, and many fruits that are also sweet—pears, apples, etc. Vinegar can be both sour and bitter. Sour foods obstruct movement so are useful for combating diarrhea and excessive sweating.

BITTER FOODS

These include lettuce, asparagus, hops, coffee, and celery and are generally cooling to reduce body temperature and dry Body Fluids. Bitter foods can be classified as "bitter and drying" or "bitter and purging," with the latter group used in constipation.

SALTY FOODS

These obviously include salt and also various seaweeds, and are regarded as softening and descending, used to soften hardness such as swollen glandular or hardened lymph nodes.

SUBTLE FLAVORS

Within the basic five-taste model there are also subtle gradations in flavor: some foods can be very bitter, others less so. Many fruits are classified as both sweet and sour—riper and cooked fruits tend to be sweet, under-ripe and raw fruits tend to be sour. The five classic tastes are sometimes augmented by a sixth—bland or neutral—which

tends to be diuretic in action. Sweet, pungent and neutral flavors are generally regarded as *yang* while salty, bitter and sour foods are *yin* in character.

A good balance of tastes is important to maintain health and any diet that allows one to become over-dominant can lead to illness. Health is maintained by the right balance of tastes while disharmonies can be corrected by adjusting the flavor of particular meals.

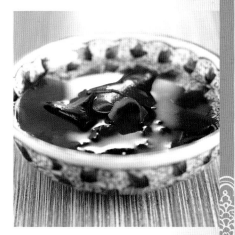

Seaweed, such as Japanese wakame, is classified as salty in Chinese theory.

FIVE ENERGIES

Foods are also defined as cold, hot, warm, cool, and neutral. These classifications have nothing to do with the actual temperature of the foods but describe their effects on the body.

COLD AND COOL FOODS

Cold foods include bamboo shoots, banana, clams, crab, grapefruit, lettuce, persimmon, seaweed, water chestnut, watercress, and watermelon while cool foods include apple, bean curd, button mushrooms, cucumber, lettuce, mango, mung beans, pear, spinach, strawberry, and tomato.

NEUTRAL FOODS

These include apricot, beef, beetroot, Chinese leaves, carrot, celery, corn (maize), egg, duck, figs, grapes, honey, polished white rice, mussels, pig's kidney, potato, pumpkin, and white sugar.

WARM AND HOT FOODS

Warm foods include brown sugar, cherry, chicken, chives, dates, spring onions, ham, kumquat, leek, mutton, peach, raspberry, prawns, walnuts, wine, and sunflower seed, while hot foods include ginger, pepper, green and red peppers, and soybean oil.

BALANCING

Foods that are heating tend to be more *yang* and drying in character whereas cooling foods are more *yin* and moistening. Too many cold or cool foods—especially during the *yin* seasons of the year—can increase Body Fluids and cause, for example, diarrhea due to Cold and Damp. Too many warm or hot foods can have a

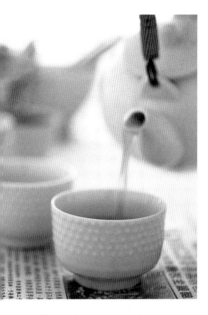

In Chinese theory green tea is more cooling than black tea.

healthy people have their own individual bias in basic constitution. Some tend to be more *yin* while others are predominantly *yang*: some also tend to feel the cold more, while others tend to be hotter so may always feel thirsty. A hot person should tend to eat more colds foods than average to help maintain an ideal *yin-yang* balance, while someone who is always cold should opt for more warming dishes. Eating a little more of the foods that help combat any intrinsic imbalances and disharmonies and avoiding those that emphasize such weaknesses can help to maintain good health.

reverse over-drying and over-heating effect, causing other health problems associated with Heat and Dryness.

While in ill health a Cold condition such as a chill or watery diarrhea, would be treated with warming foods, and a Hot problem, such as an inflammation with cooling food,

In the same way that tastes need to be balanced within a meal to maintain equilibrium, then so too with energies: in traditional cooking hot and cold foods are often combined to neutralize any imbalance that a surfeit of one or other may cause. This type of rebalancing is also found in Western tradition—adding pepper (hot) or summer savory (a hot herb) to beans (which are cold) for example.

FOOD MOVEMENTS

Along with tastes and energies, foods also have a direction, helping to move *qi* and Fluids through the body.

UP/DOWN, INWARD/OUTWARD

Solid, heavy foods such as roots will fall or sink, while lighter foods such as leaves will encourage energy to rise or float. Foods that encourage downward motion can help to relieve vomiting and hiccoughs, while foods that encourage upward movement can be useful for diarrhea or prolapse.

Foods that encourage energy flows outward may increase perspiration and have a cooling effect in fevers, while foods that encourage inward movement may be appropriate in diarrhea or abdominal discomfort.

Hen's eggs come into the category of "rising/upward" foods.

In general, meals need to contain a balance of these various types of foods to ensure that the over-all effect is neutral. Occasionally,

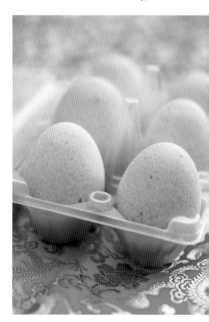

however, a specific direction may be needed: coughs or nausea associated with rising or Rebellious *qi*, for example, can be helped by foods that encourage the downward motion of *qi* while chronic constipation could be helped by foods encouraging outward motion. Foods that are upward and outward are better in spring and summer, while those that are inward and down are better in autumn and winter.

Rising/upward foods: these include aduki bean, apricot, bean, beetroot, black fungus, Chinese leaves, carrots, celery, cow's milk, duck, figs, grapes, hen's eggs, honey, hyacinth beans, kidney beans, olives, pineapple, pork, potato, shiitake mushroom, sweet potato, and white sugar.

Falling/downward foods: these include apple, eggplant, bamboo shoots, banana, bean curd, button mushrooms, grapefruit, kumquat, Job's tears, lettuce, mango, mung beans, peach, strawberry, tangerine, water chestnut, and wheat.

Outward foods: these include black pepper, ginger, green and red pepper, and soybean oil.

Inward foods: these include crab, lettuce, seaweeds.

COMBINING FOODS

While ensuring that each meal contains the correct mixture of tastes, energies and movements to ensure balance, foods can also be cooked together to neutralize the effects of their dominant characteristics. Crab, for example, is a very *yin* food, salty and cold. It is often served in western Chinese restaurants with sweet corn added, a *yang* food that helps to neutralize the *yin* tendencies and there may be a pinch of *zi si ye* (perilla leaf), a warm and pungent herb, added to the dish as well. Without the sweet corn and the perilla leaf, a very *yin* individual would be likely to suffer from diarrhea and stomach cramps due to the cold crab—with it the food is quite safe.

EATING IN SEASON

The ancient Taoists believed in being at one with their environment by eating foods to match the seasons. In 21st-century society, however, we tend to be insulated from the extremes of seasonal change. Air conditioning and central heating mean that we are rarely subjected to temperature extremes considered normal to the ancient Chinese.

The idea of eating Cold foods as we move from centrally heated home, to car, to office in the depths of winter, in order to be more in tune with our frosty environment seems rather less relevant. Instead of trying to chill our internal body region so that it matches the outside temperature we are more likely to need to maintain a steady state throughout the year.

TASTE, SEASON AND ZANG-FU ORGANS

Element	Wood	Fire	Earth	Metal	Water
Taste	Sour	Bitter	Sweet	Pungent/acrid	Salty
Season	Spring	Summer	Late Summer	Autumn	Winter
Solid or *zang* organs	Liver	Heart	Spleen	Lung	Kidney
Hollow or *fu* organs	Gall Bladder	Small Intestine	Stomach	Large Intestine	Urinary Bladder

Tastes are, however, related to the seasons and provide a more practicable guide to the right foods to eat at the right times.

Seasonal change in the *yin* and *yang* balance is also important when it comes to choosing foods. In spring the weather tends to be changeable and so food needs to be neutral to help the body cope with the sudden changes in climate. Dishes should be neither predominantly cooling nor over-stimulating.

In contrast, summer is a very *yang* time so cooling meals are needed to support *yin*: less meat with more vegetables and fish dishes are ideal. Oily, fatty foods should be avoided and alcoholic intake limited since this is heating. In autumn the weather starts to become more *yin* again, so it is a time for warmer dishes with more meat and less of the very *yin* fruits. In winter the weather is cold and so is the body, so it is time for heating foods: more alcohol and Hot meats such as lamb and chicken.

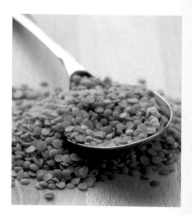

In Europe red lentils are often used in warming soups and stews.

As well as eating good-quality seasonal food, matched to constitution and needs, a healthy diet should also include regular, moderate meals. The Chinese never eat to full capacity and space their meals regularly through the day. Traditionally, breakfast—usually a rice or noodle dish with steamed buns—is taken at 6 am, with a substantial lunch at 12 noon and the evening meal at 6 pm. In between there are likely to be assorted snacks of rice noodles or *dim sum*—tasty nibbles—enjoyed mid-morning.

SPRING

Associated with Wind, spring is a time of upheaval, change and cleansing when energies tend to move upward. Some Chinese therapists recommend a period of semi-fasts with only fruit and vegetable juices at this time of year.

The over-all balance of meals needs to be neutral rather than overly heating or cooling. As well as seasonal foods, meals at this time of year should include:

- **beans:** lentils, kidney beans, peas
- **grains:** wheat, barley, oats, rye
- **seasonal fruits and vegetables:** carrots, celery, potatoes, early salad greens, asparagus and young vegetables, citrus fruits, sprouted seeds
- **meat:** chicken, pork, duck, beef

Dishes should be lightly stir-fried rather than the heavier roasts and casseroles associated with winter.

Cleansing fruit fasts are often recommended in the spring.

SPRING VEGETABLE STIR-FRY

Serves 4

2 tablespoons olive oil or
  walnut oil
12 oz (375 g) asparagus, cut
  into 2 inch (5 cm) pieces
12 oz (375 g) mangetout
bunch of spring onions, chopped
1 tablespoon raspberry vinegar
2 tablespoons chopped mint
2 tablespoons finely chopped
  chives

Eating plenty of fresh, young vegetables in spring is a good way to cleanse the body after the dark days of winter. Asparagus is bitter and warm to restimulate the digestion while spring onions help to disperse Cold, strengthen *qi* and warm the Stomach. Early sprigs of mint and the first chives from the garden will add to the flavor and help provide warming *yang* herbs as the weather starts to change.

Heat a wok, add the oil and stir-fry the asparagus and mangetout for 2 minutes; then add the chopped spring onions. Remove from the heat and toss in the raspberry vinegar, mint, and chives.

Garnish with sprigs of mint and serve with crusty French bread for lunch.

SUMMER

Summer is associated with Heat and *yang*. In Chinese theory there is also a short period called late summer which traditionally lasts for one month when the temperatures soar. Late summer is also associated with dampness. Both are periods of high energy when the Fire element prevails and when energy moves outward.

Over-stimulating and warming foods such as coffee, alcohol, red meats, and fatty foods should be avoided, with the emphasis on floating or outward-moving foods such as spices, flowers, and leaves. As well as seasonal foods, meals at this time of year should include:

- **beans:** mung beans, aduki beans, red and green lentils, chickpeas
- **grains:** corn, millet, barley
- **fresh herbs:** basil, coriander, mint

- **seasonal fruits and vegetables:** cucumbers, peppers, tomatoes, bitter salad greens (including endive and watercress), spring onions, chives, strawberries, raspberries, apricots, peaches, with apples, squash, and eggplant in late summer
- **fish/meat:** most sea fish as well as oysters, clams, crab, carp, chicken, tuna, eggs
- **pungent spices:** curry, pepper, garlic, ginger

Dishes should be lightly cooked, served cold, involve boiling rather than roasting or include raw salad ingredients.

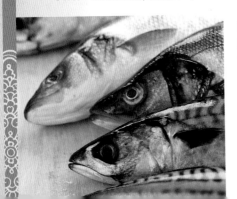

Most types of sea fish are cooling and make ideal food for hot summer days.

RED MULLET WITH TOMATO

Serves 4

2 shallots, finely chopped
1 garlic clove, crushed
1 tablespoon olive oil
12 oz (375 g) passata or a can
    of crushed Italian tomatoes
1 level teaspoon ground
    coriander seeds
1 teaspoon chopped thyme
a pinch of sugar
1 tablespoon shredded basil
8 red mullet fillets, or four
    whole red mullet, filleted
    and pin-boned, skin on
seasoned flour
1 tablespoon olive oil
salt and freshly ground black
    pepper, to taste

Tomatoes are intrinsically cooling and complemented in this sauce by pungent herbs that are also stimulating and energizing. The fish is more neutral-to-cool with a salty taste.

Heat the oven to 325°F/160°C.

Sauté the shallots and garlic in the olive oil in a saucepan. Pour in the passata or chopped tomatoes and add the coriander, thyme, sugar, and salt and pepper. Cover the pan and simmer over a low heat for 30 minutes, stirring occasionally to avoid burning or sticking, to produce a thick sauce that should not be at all watery. Add the basil at the end of the cooking time.

Coat the red mullet fillets in seasoned flour and fry gently in the tablespoon of olive oil for 1–2 minutes each side. Transfer the fillets to a serving dish and spoon over the tomato sauce. Cook in the preheated oven for 10 minutes.

Allow to cool to room temperature and serve with a green salad.

AUTUMN

In China autumn is associated with dryness. Temperatures are starting to fall and traditional Chinese cooking for this time of year tends to focus on foods to "lubricate the intestines" to combat seasonal dryness.

Energy moves downward in the autumn so root vegetables are eaten to encourage this downward motion. As well as seasonal foods, meals at this time of year should include:

- **beans:** soybeans, tofu, and other soy products
- **grains:** rice, wild rice, barley, wheat
- **seasonal fruits and vegetables:** cabbage, bamboo shoots, cauliflower, pumpkin, winter squash, spinach, water chestnuts, apples, pears, mangoes, kumquats
- **meat and fish:** cod, salmon, chicken, turkey

Dishes should move gradually toward the roast meats and casseroles associated with winter.

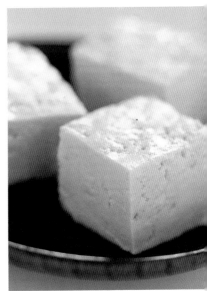

Soybean curd or tofu has been eaten in China for more than 1,000 years.

PUMPKIN AND WATER CHESTNUT RISOTTO

Serves 4

3 tablespoons olive oil
1 small pumpkin, skin and seeds
  removed, chopped
1½ pints (1 liter) vegetable
  stock
2 oz (50 g) unsalted butter
1 leek, finely sliced
2 garlic cloves, crushed
10 oz (300 g) risotto rice,
  such as arborio or vialone
8 oz (250 g) can water
  chestnuts, drained and halved
  or 8 fresh water chestnuts,
  peeled and sliced
1 tablespoon chopped thyme

Pumpkin is sweet and warm so helps to strengthen the Spleen and replenish *qi*. This is balanced by the water chestnuts, which are also sweet but Cold in nature. They encourage the production of Body Fluids and help strengthen Lung *yin* so are ideal for the dry coughs and wheezes common as the weather changes in autumn. Thyme is a warming herb and specific for the Lungs.

Heat 2 tablespoons of oil in a frying pan and sauté the pumpkin for about 15 minutes or until it is soft. Heat the vegetable stock in a separate saucepan so that is gently simmering: keep it hot.

Melt the butter in a large pan, add the remaining oil and sauté the thinly sliced leek. When it is soft add the crushed garlic and rice and stir for 2 minutes until the rice is sticky and coated with the oil and butter. Slowly add the hot vegetable stock, a ladle at a time, while constantly stirring the rice mixture.

After about 15 minutes add the cooked pumpkin chunks to the risotto and continue cooking until the rice is *al dente* and all the stock is absorbed. Add the water chestnuts during the final 5 minutes of cooking, and heat thoroughly. Serve sprinkled with the fresh thyme.

WINTER

Winter is cold with *yin* dominating: dark, damp, cold. Moving from autumn to winter is another major seasonal change when we need to eat plenty of energizing herbs and preventatives to combat the increased risk of external pathogens in the months ahead. It is a time when energy moves inward—supported by grains, seeds, and nuts.

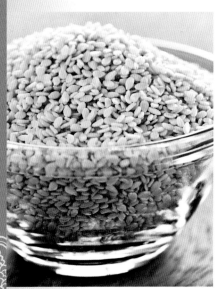

In China sesame seeds are roasted to make sesame seed oil (*zhi ma you*).

As well as seasonal foods, meals at this time of year should include:

- **beans:** kidney beans. aduki beans, black beans, pinto beans
- **grains:** brown rice, wheat, barley, millet, oats
- **seeds:** sesame, sunflower
- **seasonal fruits and vegetables:** carrots, parsnips, turnips, onions, potatoes, cranberries
- **meat and fish:** halibut, salmon, beef, lamb
- **pungent herbs and spices:** including garlic, ginger, pepper, thyme, rosemary

The emphasis should be on roasting and baking: roast meats, stews, and casseroles.

OAT PORRIDGE WITH CINNAMON AND GOJI BERRIES

Serves 4

butter
8 oz (250 g) medium oatmeal or porridge oats
1 pint (600 ml) soy or cow's milk
1 tablespoon maple syrup
1 oz (25 g) goji berries (gou qi zi)
$\frac{1}{2}$ teaspoon cinnamon powder
2 oz (50 g) sunflower seeds
1 oz (25 g) black sesame seeds
pinch of salt

Oats are a stimulating food for the nervous system, energizing and anti-depressant. They are a rich source of B vitamins, they lower cholesterol levels, help to regulate blood sugar and contain iron and iodine. Gou qi zi, sold as goji berries, help to nourish Blood and tonify Liver and Kidneys. Cinnamon helps to clear internal cold and warm the Kidneys.

Heat the oven to 375°F/190°C.

Using the butter, generously grease a glass or ceramic ovenproof dish.

Put the oatmeal, milk, maple syrup, goji berries, cinnamon, sunflower seeds, sesame seeds, and salt into the dish. Mix well and place in the preheated oven for 30 minutes. Check the porridge and stir after 15 minutes and add a little more hot water or milk if it is sticking or becoming too thick and solid.

Serve with crème fraîche, cream, or warm milk as desired.

USEFUL CHINESE FOOD INGREDIENTS

Hyacinth bean (*bai biandou*): Used to strengthen the Spleen *qi*, regulate Stomach function and remove excess Heat, Damp, and Phlegm.

Ginkgo nut (*bai guo*): The seeds of the ginkgo tree are popular in Chinese vegetarian cookery; medicinally they help to consolidate Lung *qi* and relieve asthma. Eaten raw they are a folk remedy for hangovers.

Water chestnut (*bi qi*): A cooling food that is also nourishing for Spleen and Stomach. Water chestnuts are traditionally given as a purgative to children who have swallowed coins.

Winter melon (*dong gua*): A gourd rather than a melon, which despite its name is a summer vegetable. The peel and seeds are sweet and cool and used to clear Heat, mainly from Spleen and Lung, and relieve thirst. The flesh of the melon is used in folk medicine to cool fevers and as a diuretic; chewing the seeds is believed to suppress hunger and prolong life.

Bean curd (*doufu*): Known as tofu in the West, this has been made in China at least since the Tang Dynasty (618–907CE). It is a rich source of protein and vitamins and is easily digestible. Tofu is sweet and cool and acts on Spleen, Stomach, and Large Intestine. It is said to invigorate *qi*, increase Body Fluids and clear Heat and Toxins.

Sweet potato (*gan shu*): Sweet potato is considered to be a strength-giving food especially beneficial for Spleen, Stomach, and Kidney.

Chinese red dates or jujube (*hong zao*): In folk tradition red dates are considered to be strengthening in debility and convalescence. They are used in numerous dishes. Medicinally, they replenish Spleen and Stomach *qi* and nourish Blood.

Bitter melon (*ku gua*): A gourd rather than a melon, it is used to stimulate the digestion and as a cooling remedy in fevers. Bitter melon is used as a folk remedy for malaria and as a *yang* tonic. Recent research suggests the plant may also strengthen the immune system.

Lotus root *(lianou):* Despite growing in muddy water the lotus is traditionally regarded as a symbol of purity and is used as a cleansing remedy and to rid the body of poisons. The root (often stir-fried as a vegetable) helps to strengthen the Spleen, aids the digestion and also replenishes Blood. The seeds are eaten as a sweet snack in summer or dried and made into a paste for use in cake fillings; these tonify Spleen, Stomach, and Kidney and are sedative.

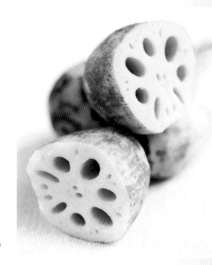

Lotus root has a mild sweet flavor and a crunchy texture.

Longan *(long yan rou)* and **lychee** *(lizhi):* Both are popular fruits in China, longan are raisin-like fruits that nourish the Blood and tonify Heart and Spleen. They are a smaller relation of the more familiar lychee, which is used to ease thirst and, in folk remedies, for swollen glands; the pips are believed to invigorate *qi* and relieve abdominal Cold and pain.

Chinese radish (*luo bo*): Used to stimulate the appetite and crushed in poultices for burns and bruises. Radishes are traditionally believed by the Chinese to treat insanity and warts.

Mango *(mang gua):* Mangoes are traditionally eaten to relieve thirst and they can also improve the circulation and regulate menstruation. Mangoes are a good source of vitamin A.

Rice *(mi* or *jing mi)*: Boiled rice gruel is the basis for many therapeutic dishes for treating digestive disorders and is considered an ideal food for the elderly and very young. Rice flour and rice noodles are used in many dishes. Glutinous rice is a sweeter form of rice regarded as a luxury and used in dishes for special occasions. Rice is used medicinally to replenish Spleen and Stomach *qi*

Eggplant has been eaten in China since at least the third century CE.

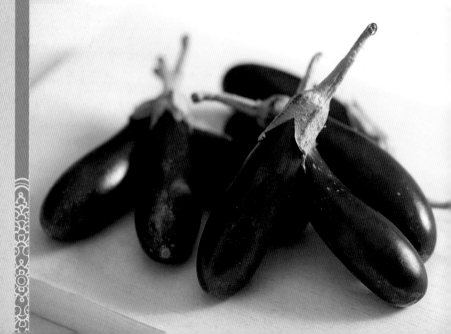

while rice sprouts help to clear food stagnation and improve the digestion. Rice vinegar (*mi cu*) improves the digestion, it is used for coughs and influenza and as a preventative for epidemic disease.

Black fungus or wood ear/*Auricularia auricula* (*mu er* or *hei mu er*):

A rich source of minerals, black fungus is also believed to reduce the risk of heart attacks and inhibit blood clots. It is an effective immune tonic that also helps replenish *jīng*, move Blood, cleanse the womb and ease excessive menstrual bleeding. It is more therapeutic than cloud ear fungus, also known as black fungus *Auricularia polytricha*. The fungus is usually sold dried and must be soaked in warm water for up to 30 minutes before use.

Eggplant (*qiè zi*):

Regarded as cooling and used with vinegar in poultices for abscesses. The burned stalks are used in folk medicine for hemorrhoids and toothache.

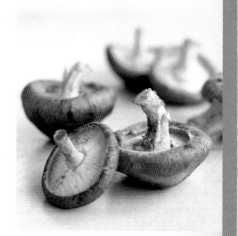

Shiitake mushrooms are known to stimulate the immune system and protect the Liver.

Shiitake mushrooms/*Lentinus edodes* (*xiang fu*):

These have been shown in modern research to be an effective immune stimulant with proven anti-viral action; they contain essential amino acids, are anti-tumor and protective for the Liver, Shiitake mushrooms also soothe bronchial inflammations and normalize digestion in *Candida* infections. Traditionally they are used to tonify *qi* and Blood.

White fungus/*Tremella fuciformis* (*yin er, xue er* or *bai mu*): An important *yin* tonic that is also taken for insomnia, Liver, and Lung problems and chronic constipation. The fungus is usually sold dried and must be soaked in warm water for up to 30 minutes before use.

Job's tears (*yi yi ren*): This cereal is rich in nutrients (especially B vitamins) and amino acids. When cooked it becomes soft and mucilaginous and is easily digested— it is generally used in soups as an alternative to barley. It is a good tonic for the Spleen, and is used for diarrhea, to clear Damp, and regulate water metabolism.

Sweet corn *(yumi):* Corn is eaten regularly by some as a Heart tonic and to enhance sexual capacity. A decoction of the root and leaves is a folk remedy for urinary problems.

Taro *(yu tou):* A root vegetable generally eaten as dumplings or cakes in *dim sum*. The seeds of the taro are used for indigestion and the leaves and stalks for insect bites.

Bamboo shoots (*zhu sun*): While the shoots are used in cooking the sap shavings and leaves of the black bamboo are used medicinally to clear Phlegm and Heat in the Lung and Stomach. The leaf is a longstanding folk remedy for tuberculosis.

HERBS, SPICES, AND FLAVORINGS

Five-spice powder: A popular flavoring combination largely used in restaurants and the West rather than domestic Chinese cuisine. The five-spice mix typically contains Sichuan peppercorns (*hua jiao*), star anise (*ba jiao*), Chinese cinnamon (*rou gui*), cloves (*ding xiang*), fennel seeds (*xiao hui xiang*). Anise seed (*Pimpinella anisum*) and ginger root (*jiang*) are sometimes substituted for the fennel and Sichuan peppercorns.

Star anise (*ba jiao*): Used in five-spice powder (see above) as a popular seasoning, it is a warming remedy for abdominal pain associated with Cold and helps to regulate *qi* circulation. It is used in folk medicine for lumbago and urinary complaints and is added as a flavoring to cough mixtures.

Tangerine peel (*chen pi*): This medicinal herb is widely used as a seasoning in meat dishes.

Spring onion (*cong bai* or *qing cong*): Used to encourage sweating in chills and fevers and eaten for catarrh, headaches, and diarrhea. Also given to children as a sedative and used in poultices for abscesses and fractures. It disperses Cold by invigorating *yang qi* and eases abdominal fullness.

Chinese cinnamon (*gui*): The peel or fine bark (*rou gui*) is used in cooking as well as the thicker rolls of bark (*gui pi*). Cinnamon is a warming remedy good for chills which also tonifies the Kidneys.

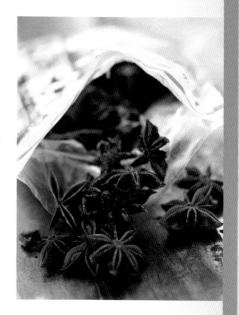

Star anise is an ingredient of five-spice powder widely used in the West.

Black sesame (*hei zhi ma*): This is used for Deficient Liver and Kidney *yin*, to nourish Blood and lubricate the digestive system.

Sichuan peppercorns (*hua jiao*, *chuan jiao* or *ye shan jiao*): While the berries are an important culinary ingredient, both the leaves and

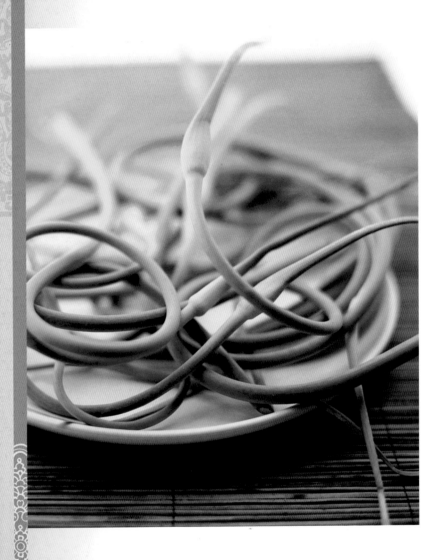

berries are also used for digestive problems, especially Spleen and Stomach deficiency with abdominal pain, vomiting, and diarrhea. The root is taken for Kidney and Urinary Bladder weakness. The bark is used to warm Spleen and Stomach and relieve pain due to Cold. It is one of the ingredients of Chinese five-spice powder (see above).

Black and white pepper (*hu jiao*): Ground white pepper is most commonly used in Chinese cooking. It is added in large quantities to dishes for colds, influenza, dysentery, and vomiting.

Ginger (*jiang*): Ginger is widely used in Chinese medicine as a warming remedy to combat Wind Cold: in cooking ginger helps to neutralize Cold foods and warm the *middle jiao* to combat nausea.

Chinese chives (*ju cai*): Also known as garlic chives. Believed to nourish

and purify Blood and act as a general tonic in debility. They are used as a folk remedy for dog, snake, and insect bites.

Garlic (*suan*): Used for Spleen, Stomach and Kidneys and to neutralize the effects of toxic ingredients.

Coriander (*yan shi*): A stimulating and cleansing herb used to remove toxins and carminative to ease indigestion.

Chinese chives have a subtle garlic flavor and are an ideal flavoring for egg dishes.

ENERGIZING FOODS

In Chinese theory our vital energy—*qi*—is composed of primordial *qi* derived from our parents; nature *qi* from the air we breathe and grain *qi* from the food we eat. Grain *qi* is also largely responsible for nourishing *qi*, which is a source of Blood, and contributes toward pectoral *qi* which controls respiration and heartbeat.

Given the vital role of grain *qi*, it is clear that good food is essential to maintain vital energy. *Qi* tonics, such as *ren shen* (Korean ginseng), *huang qi* (milk vetch root), and *dang shen* (bellflower root), can be added to dishes to provide energy-giving meals: simply add a small piece of the roots to stews and casseroles, which can be removed before serving or eaten with the meal.

Other foods are intrinsically energy giving and are worth eating regularly. Quail's eggs (*chunniaodan*), for example, are known in the East as "animal ginseng." They are neutral in character with a sweet flavor, invigorate *qi*, replenish Blood and strengthen the muscles and bones. They are an excellent energy-giving food for the elderly and are especially helpful for those suffering from arthritis, lumbago, or weakness in the lower limbs. They can be eaten hard-boiled in salads or eaten for breakfast instead of hen's eggs.

Quail's eggs are known as "animal ginseng" in the East and make a good alternative to hen's eggs.

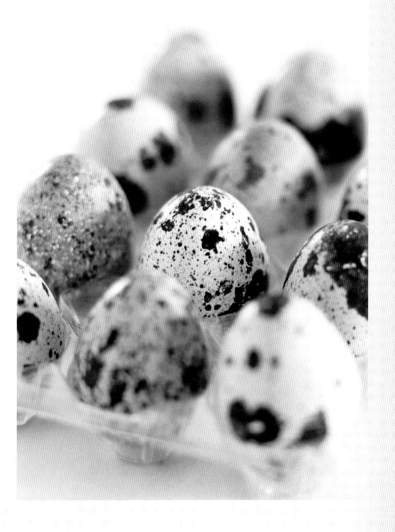

SIX TREASURES CHICKEN SOUP

Serves 4–6

2 spring onions, chopped

$1/2$ inch (1 cm) piece fresh ginger root, peeled and chopped

2 garlic cloves, crushed

2 tablespoons sherry or rice wine

1 tablespoon soy sauce

1 tablespoon sesame oil

2 teaspoons sugar

8 chicken thighs

$1/3$ oz (10 g) milk vetch (*huang qi*)

$1/3$ oz (10 g) Chinese yam (*shan yao*)

$1/3$ oz (10 g) Chinese angelica (*dang gui*)

$1/3$ oz (10 g) Solomon's seal root (*yu zhu*)

$1/3$ oz (10 g) eucommia bark (*du zhong*)

10 pieces black Chinese dates (*da zao*)

3 dried shiitake mushrooms, soaked in hot water for 10 minutes

1 small can water chestnuts, drained

1–2 tablespoons chopped coriander leaves, to garnish

This combination of herbs and chicken nourishes the Blood, improves Blood circulation, strengthens *qi* and Kidney *yang*, and nourishes Kidney *yin*. The soup is good for exhaustion, low libido and to strengthen immunity. The method of steaming the chicken in a covered clay pot with other tonic herbs for up to 10 hours is popular in China and is believed to enhance the healing properties. In China the chicken is discarded although it is still good to eat. Soups like this are generally served before a meal in Southern China or after a meal with steamed bread in Northern China.

Heat the oven to 300°F/150°C

Mix together the spring onions, ginger, garlic, sherry, sesame oil, sugar, and soy sauce and marinate the chicken pieces for two hours. Place the chicken pieces, herbs and shiitake in a clay pot and cover with boiling water. Cover and cook in the oven for 6 hours.

Add the water chestnuts in the last 20 minutes.

Strain the soup and remove the chicken bones then add the chicken thigh meat, shiitake, water chestnuts and black dates to the liquid, discard the rest of the herbs, and heat gently to warm through. Serve sprinkled with chopped coriander.

BEAN CURD WITH QUAILS' EGGS AND CHINESE CHIVES

Serves 4

One pack of bean curd (tofu)
    cut into $\frac{1}{2}$ inch (1 cm) cubes
8 quails' eggs, beaten
a handful of finely chopped
    Chinese chives
salt and black pepper, to season
knob of butter
1–2 tablespoons olive oil
1 spring onion, finely chopped
4 oz (125 g) mung bean sprouts
2 fl oz (50 ml) vegetable stock
1 tablespoon rice wine

Quails' eggs and bean curd (tofu) are both
energy-giving foods while bean curd also
combats the toxic effects of sulphur (from
pollution) and alcohol, by removing poisons and
excreting excess Heat in the urine. Fresh bean
curd will keep for several days if covered in
water and stored in the refrigerator.

Boil the bean curd in a pan of water for
2–3 minutes to harden, remove from the heat
and drain. Mix the beaten eggs with half the
chives and salt and pepper. Melt the butter in a
small pan and scramble the egg mixture for
1–2 minutes until lightly cooked.

In a wok heat the olive oil and stir-fry the bean
curd, spring onion and bean sprouts for
2 minutes until the bean sprouts are slightly
translucent. Add the stock and rice wine, bring
to the boil and simmer for 3–4 minutes. Add
the scrambled eggs, sprinkle with the remaining
chives and serve immediately with a green salad
for lunch.

FOODS TO STRENGTHEN THE DIGESTION

A strong and efficient digestive system is seen as vital to good health in all cultures: Ayurvedic medicine regards *agni* (digestive fire) almost as a deity; while medieval European doctors argued that "death dwells in the bowels." In Chinese medicine Spleen and Stomach are not only responsible for digestion but also have responsibility for controlling Blood, managing the upward flow of *qi* and storing determination.

Spleen and Stomach weakness can manifest as a wide range of digestive upsets—from indigestion to constipation—as well as being associated with poor memory and mental confusion. The *san jiao* (Triple Burner) also plays a vital role in good digestion; weakness and deficiency here is likely to upset *qi* movements and distribution of the *wèi qi* (defence energy).

Foods for the digestive system include dishes cooked with strengthening herbs as well as easy-to-eat grains such as *yi yi ren* (Job's tear seeds). Rice is regarded as especially valuable for a wide range of digestive disorders and is often made into therapeutic gruel or porridge usually known as congee.

Rice is widely used a therapeutic food often made into either a thin gruel or a thicker porridge or congee.

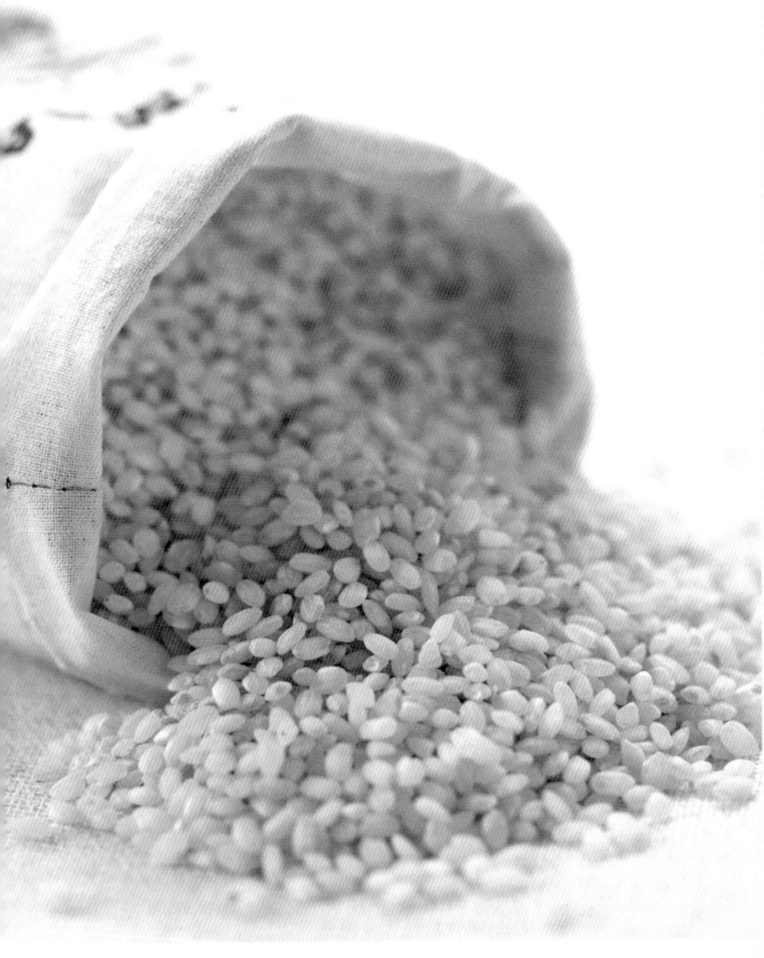

RICE PORRIDGE WITH YI YI REN AND BEANS

Serves 6

1 oz (25 g) red kidney beans
  (tinned or fresh)
4 oz (125 g) round grain rice
½ oz (15 g) Job's tear seeds
  (*yi yi ren*)
½ oz (15 g) hyacinth bean
  (*bian biandou*)
1¾ pints (1 liter) water or
  vegetable stock
bunch of spring onions or
  flat-leaved parsley, chopped,
  to garnish (optional)

This porridge is ideal for those suffering from weak, sluggish digestion. It can be served as a light supper dish, for lunch or breakfast. Kidney beans (*Phaseolus vulgaris*) originated in South America but by the 16th century had spread to Asia, and China is now one of the world's most significant growers of the crop. They are high in protein, vitamins, and minerals (including iron) and also help to stabilize blood sugar levels. *Yi yi ren* and hyacinth beans both help to strengthen the Spleen and remove excess Damp and Phlegm.

If using fresh kidney beans, wash and cover with water and leave to soak overnight; drain, rinse and cover with fresh water, then bring to the boil, boiling vigorously for 45–50 minutes before straining. With tinned beans simply drain and rinse thoroughly in water.

To the prepared beans, add the rice, Job's tear seeds, hyacinth beans and water or stock in a large saucepan, cover with water and simmer for 45–60 minutes. The rice grains will absorb most of the water and burst to produce a thick porridge. Add more water or stock during cooking if need be. Serve in soup bowls and garnish with spring onions or parsley as preferred.

FISH SOUP WITH LOTUS ROOT AND TANGERINE PEEL

Serves 4—6

1 fresh lotus root (or pre-cooked tinned lotus root)
2 lb (1 kg) mixed fresh fish as available, cleaned but left on the bone (use firm fish such as red mullet, monkfish or halibut)
2 tablespoons olive oil
2 onions, peeled and chopped
1 leek, thinly sliced
1 inch (2.5 cm) slice fresh ginger root, peeled and finely chopped
3 garlic cloves, peeled and sliced
2 carrots, diced
2 celery stalks, sliced
6 fresh shiitake mushrooms, sliced
1 lb (500 g) tomatoes skinned, deseeded, and chopped (or use 1 can of organic chopped tomatoes)
6 Chinese black dates (*da zao*)
2–3 pieces of tangerine peel (*chen pi*)
chopped parsley, to garnish

This soup strengthens the digestion and replenishes *qi* and Blood.

If using fresh lotus root, peel and slice the root diagonally and place in a saucepan with 1 pint (600 ml) of water, bring to the boil and simmer, covered, for two hours.

Wash the fish and cut into thick pieces cutting through the bone. Sauté gently in a little olive oil in a wok for three or four minutes until the fish is opaque and cooked through. Remove from the wok and keep warm.

Sauté the onions, leeks, ginger and garlic in the wok in a little olive oil over a very gentle heat for 10 minutes, do not allow to brown. Add the carrots, celery and shiitake to the wok and cook until soft; then add the tomatoes and simmer gently for 10 minutes over a low heat. Add the dates and tangerine peel and simmer gently for 1–2 minutes to blend the flavors.

Finally add water to the cooked lotus root and its cooking water to bring the volume back up to 1 pint (600 ml) and add this to the soup mixture; simmer for 20 minutes. Stir in the chunks of fish. Serve the soup in bowls and garnish with chopped parsley.

FOODS TO CLEAR PHLEGM AND DAMP

Phlegm is one of common causes of internal disease in Chinese medicine: it can be visible, as in the sputum from coughs; or invisible and able to collect anywhere in the body. Phlegm can be both a cause and an effect of disease.

Spleen *qi* Deficiency, for example, can cause a build-up of Phlegm as the Spleen fails to manage the water transport mechanism. Phlegm itself can then block channels or accumulate and damage other *zang-fu* organs.

Damp is one of the external pathogens that can cause disease: some people are more susceptible to Damp than others, especially if there is an underlying Spleen weakness. "Damp" people have a tendency to put on weight easily and commonly suffer from catarrhal problems.

Foods that help to tonify the Spleen can be helpful in Phlegm conditions. The Spleen is associated with the Earth element and the taste "sweet;" foods in this category include cooked carrots, sweet potatoes, sweet corn, banana, swedes, parsnips, celery, and tomatoes (both also with a sour taste), leeks, onions, sweet rice, butter, beef, chicken, chicken liver, cooked peaches, honey, maple syrup, and unrefined sugars.

Sweet foods, such as honey, can often help to tonify the Spleen.

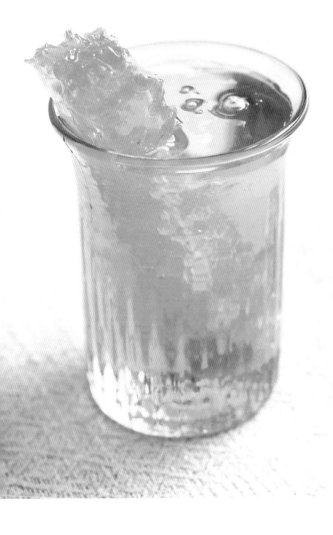

BEEF STIR-FRY WITH TANGERINE PEEL

Serves 4

1 tablespoon tangerine peel
(*chen pi*), finely sliced
4 oz (125 g) carrots, very finely
sliced
4 oz (125 g) leeks, finely sliced
1/2 tablespoon olive oil
1 lb (500 g) beef fillet pieces,
cut into thin strips
1 tablespoon seasoned flour
1 garlic clove, crushed
1 teaspoon chopped ginger root
pinch of sugar
1 small glass rice wine or dry
sherry
8 fl oz (250 ml) of vegetable,
beef or chicken stock
1 teaspoon arrowroot or corn
flour, stirred into a paste with
a little water
salt and pepper, to taste

This warming dish helps to clear excess Damp and Phlegm while the tangerine peel is a good tonic for the Spleen and helps to regulate its action. Tangerine peel (*chen pi*) is easy to make at home by drying the peel of organically grown tangerines and storing for several weeks before using. Chinese therapeutic meals should be cooked with as little oil as possible—if you have a non-stick pan it is usually possible to dry-fry meats although vegetables may need a little oil to improve the cooking.

Soak a piece of tangerine peel in a cup of boiling water for 5–10 minutes to soften, then cut into very fine slices.

Sauté the carrots and leeks in the olive oil until they start to soften. Toss the beef slices in the seasoned flour, then add to the pan with the garlic, ginger, tangerine peel and a pinch of sugar. Cook for about 3–4 minutes until the meat is browned (longer if you prefer it well cooked), then add the rice wine or sherry and bubble vigorously for a couple of minutes.

Add the stock and thicken with the arrowroot or cornflour mixture. Bring to the boil. Season with salt and pepper to taste if required and serve on a bed of boiled rice.

SALMON AND WAKAME WITH BUCKWHEAT NOODLES

Serves 2

2 shiitake mushrooms, sliced
2 inch (5 cm) piece ginger root,
    peeled and finely chopped
2 spring onions, chopped
2 shallots, finely sliced
1 garlic clove, crushed
1 tablespoon sesame oil
1 tablespoon soy sauce
10 fl oz (300 ml) fish stock
1 oz (25 g) dried wakame
    seaweed
1 tablespoon rice wine
5 oz (150 g) buckwheat noodles
2 salmon fillets, skinned

Wakame seaweed (*Undaria pinnatifida*) is readily available in supermarkets and Chinese stores where it is called *qundaicai*. It nourishes *yin* and helps to transforms Phlegm. It is also cooling for Hot conditions and is used here with warming herbs, ginger and garlic.

If using dried shiitake soak the mushrooms in warm water for 10–15 minutes before slicing.

In a hot wok stir-fry the ginger, spring onions, shallots and garlic in a little of the sesame oil for 2 minutes, add a teaspoon of the soy sauce and put to one side to keep warm.

Stir-fry the shiitake in a little more sesame oil for 1 minute. Heat the fish stock to just below boiling, remove from the heat and add the wakame and rice wine. Cook the buckwheat noodles in boiling water as directed on the packet and strain. While the noodles are cooking, brush the salmon fillets with soy sauce and cook under a hot grill for 3–5 minutes on each side until cooked.

Divide the noodles between two soup bowls and pour over the hot stock with the wakame. Top with the mushrooms and the salmon fillets and finally garnish with the garlic and ginger.

FOODS TO CONTROL LIVER QI

Liver *qi* disorders are commonplace with symptoms ranging from menstrual irregularities or cervical dysplasia associated with constrained Liver *qi*; headaches and insomnia linked to over-exuberant Liver *yang*, or the sore eyes and irritability associated with the flaring of Liver Fire. Cooling *yin* foods can help with excess Liver Heat or *yang* with Liver tonics used for Constrained *qi* problems.

The liver is the body's first line of defence, checking and filtering the products of digestion to remove any potentially harmful substances. In a polluted world heavily dependent on artificial pesticides and fertilizers, our food inevitably contains many substances that end up being stored in the liver leading to stagnation—a syndrome recognized by both Western and Chinese herbalists. The Liver is associated with the Wood element in Chinese theory so is especially affected by sour-tasting foods such as apple, apricot, grapefruit, mango, celery and tomato, plum, raspberry, lemon, vinegar, duck and chicken livers.

Ju hua (chrysanthemum flower) is a popular Liver remedy in China. It is widely available in tea bags as an everyday drink.

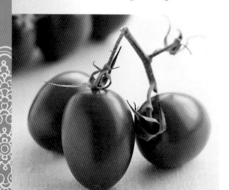

The Liver is linked with the sour taste so is helped by foods like tomatoes.

CHICKEN LIVERS AND MANGO

Serves 4

1 lb (500 g) fresh chicken livers, cut into bite-size pieces
1–2 tablespoons seasoned flour
1 tablespoon olive oil
1 tablespoon balsamic vinegar
pinch of sugar
1 ripe mango, peeled and cut into cubes
salt and freshly ground black pepper
Lettuce, young dandelion leaves, celery (shredded), spring onion (finely sliced), to serve

Chicken liver helps to ease Liver *qi* stagnation while cool and sour-tasting fresh mango controls excess Liver *yang* and Fire. Other suitable fruits such as peach, nectarines or plums can be substituted for mango in this recipe. Young dandelion leaves make a useful addition to the accompanying salad if you have them.

Toss the chicken livers in seasoned flour until well coated.

Stir-fry the chicken livers in olive oil for 5 minutes until browned on the outside but not over-cooked.

Add the balsamic vinegar, sugar, salt, and pepper and let it bubble for a minute, then remove from the heat, add the mango and mix well.

Serve on the bed of lettuce, celery and sliced spring onions: add some croutons if you like them.

FOODS TO BOOST THE IMMUNE SYSTEM

In the West, recurrent infections are often blamed on a weakened immune system. In Chinese theory the equivalent explanation would be deficient *wèi qi*, the defence energy that circulates on the skin and repels external pathogens. Tonic herbs, notably *huang qi* (milk vetch) are especially effective at strengthening *wèi qi*.

Various foods come into the immune-building category, notably mushrooms. Research in recent years has demonstrated the efficacy of many ancient Chinese remedies containing fungi. Many of these mushrooms are available in supermarkets or from specialist suppliers. They are ideal to add to therapeutic stir-fries and soups to combat seasonal chills as well as being used to support treatments for cancer and other diseases associated with weakened immunity. Worth looking out for are:

Mu huan jun (*Armillaria mellea*): Honey mushroom is sweet and cold and a nutritive tonic for Liver, Lung, Stomach, and Large Intestine.

Mu er or ***hei mu er*** (*Auricularia auricula*): Black fungus or wood ear is sweet and cool, helping to invigorate Blood and ease pain. It is also rich in amino acids, phosphorus, iron, calcium, and sugars and was traditionally used boiled in milk or beer as a remedy for throat inflammations. *Mu er* is also an effective immune tonic and replenishes *jīng* (essence).

Black fungus, also known as wood ear, is now regarded as an effective immune stimulant.

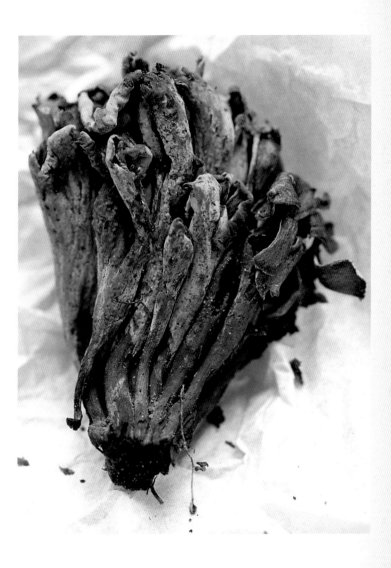

Mei wei niu gan (*Boletus edulis*): Cep mushrooms are a delicacy in both East and West; in Chinese medicine they are described as cool and salty and are an ingredient in "tendon easing pills" for lumbago and leg pains, or are cooked with pork for leukemia; they make a delicious addition to any dish.

Zhu ling (*Grifola umbellata*) and **maitake** (*Grifola frondosa*): Maitake or hen of the woods originate from Japan and have been extensively researched for their anti-tumor and immune stimulating properties; *Zhu ling* is preferred in China and is sweet and cool; it is traditionally used as a diuretic and to invigorate the Kidney.

Xiang gu (*Lentinus edodes*): Shiitake mushrooms have been studied for their immune-strengthening properties. In China they have two variant names—*dong gu* (winter mushroom) and *hua gu* (fragrant mushroom). Both are cool and sweet and are used as a strengthening and restorative remedy to tonify *qi* and Blood as well as soothing bronchial inflammations and normalizing digestion.

Hao gu (*Pleurotus ostreatus*): Oyster mushrooms are a good source of essential amino acids. They are defined as sweet and slightly warm in Chinese medicine and were traditionally used to strengthen veins, relax the tendons and dispel Cold. More recent studies have highlighted their anti-tumor properties, ability to reduce cholesterol levels in blood, and similar immune-strengthening action to shiitake mushrooms.

Ma bo (*Lasiosphaera fenslii*): Puffball is traditionally used to clear Heat and detoxify Fire Poisons. It is especially beneficial for throat problems involving swelling or laryngitis. Puffball is delicious covered in egg and breadcrumbs and fried.

REN SHEN AND HUANG QI MUSHROOM SOUP

Serves 6

1 oz (25 g) dried *hei mu er*
(hen of the woods)—or 4 oz
(125 g) fresh if available
1 onion, chopped
4 tablespoons olive oil
1¹/₂ lb (750 g) fresh shiitake or
oyster mushrooms, sliced
2 pints (1.2 liters) chicken or
vegetable stock
¹/₂ oz (15 g) Korean ginseng
(*ren shen*)
¹/₂ oz (15 g) milk vetch
(*huang qi*)
2 tablespoons créme fraîche and
chopped parsley, to garnish

If using dried *hei mu er* soak in water for
5–10 minutes to soften, then rinse in clean
water and set aside. Sauté the finely chopped
onion in the oil for 2–3 minutes until it is soft,
then add all the fresh sliced mushrooms and
continue cooking for 3 minutes.

Add the chicken or vegetable stock, ginseng,
milk vetch and pre-soaked *hei mu* (if using)
Bring to the boil, reduce the heat and simmer
for 45 minutes.

Remove from the heat and take out the pieces
of ginseng and milk vetch. Put the remainder of
the soup into a food processor or blender and
reduce to a smooth liquid.

Return to the heat and warm through before
serving, garnished with a spoonful of créme
fraîche and a little chopped parsley. The ginseng
can be chopped and served with the soup,
rather like croutons, but the milk vetch is too
fibrous to eat and should be discarded.

TIME TO DETOX

Much of the emphasis in Western dietary and nutritional regimes is on detox; the concept is largely based on the fact that Western diets contain many pollutants and that we eat too many foods that are bad for us, thus a purge is required to cleanse the system.

Traditional lifestyles and therapies had little need for these periodic detox diets since the food was healthier, less likely to be eaten in vast quantities, and prevailing culture dictated a period of fasting to provide a break from normal consumption.

This concept of a dietary "detox" is largely unknown in Chinese medicine. However, many foods are regularly consumed that do have the ability to remove toxic products from the system. Any build-up of toxins would be seen as a failure in the *zang-fu* organs to function normally and would be treated with appropriate remedies rather than depending on temporary and artificial changes in the diet.

To avoid the need to "detox" it is far better to eat healthily throughout the year ensuring a balanced diet with fresh, well-produced ingredients: locally farmed meat, fresh local vegetables, and a minimum of artificial preservatives. If you feel the need for cleansing foods then the various varieties of cabbage are well worth eating and add more ginger and coriander to your dishes as both can help cleanse the system.

Bok choy is known as *xiao bai cai* in China which translates as "little white cabbage."

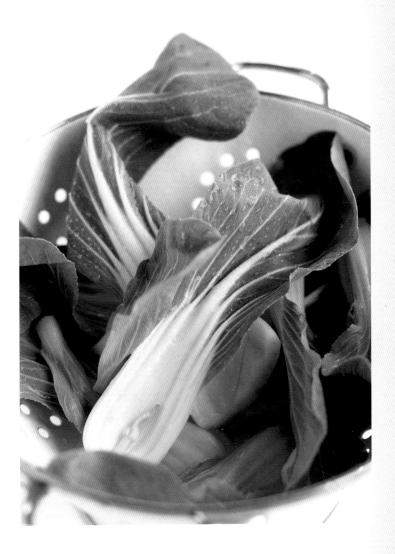

BOK CHOY IN BASIL OIL DRESSING

Serves 4

1 lb (500 g) miniature bok choy
1 tablespoon basil oil (prepared by infusing basil in olive oil for several days, or you can buy it ready-made)
Dash of chilli sauce
Dash of maple syrup
1 teaspoon crushed Sichuan peppercorns
salt, to taste

Just as cabbage is regarded in Western tradition as a cleansing and energizing remedy for the digestive system so the various Chinese greens and cabbages are used in much the same way. Bok choy is a stimulating digestive remedy which is neutral, sweet, and helpful for the Large Intestine and Stomach. In this dish it is combined with basil oil, which is also cleansing for the lower bowel and a dash of chilli, a potent anti-microbial.

Steam the bok choy for 6–7 minutes.

Meanwhile, mix the sauce ingredients together. When the bok choy is ready, toss in the dressing. Serve as a side dish or eat with bread for lunch.

FRESH CORIANDER LEAF PESTO WITH PASTA

Serves 4

1 handful fresh, organically
  grown coriander leaves, washed
6 tablespoons olive oil
1 garlic clove
2 tablespoons either almonds,
  walnuts, cashews, and/or pine
  nuts
2 tablespoons lemon juice
2 oz (50 g) feta cheese,
  crumbled
8 oz (250 g) fresh pasta such as
  spaghetti or tagliatelle
grated Parmesan cheese and
  freshly ground black pepper, to
  garnish

Coriander has become a familiar culinary herb in recent years, although as *yan shi*, it is long established in Chinese medicine as a stimulating and cleansing herb used to remove toxins. Coriander leaves are now known to accelerate the excretion of toxic metals such as mercury, lead, and aluminium from the body.

Put the coriander and olive oil in a food processor and blend until finely chopped. Add the garlic, nuts, and lemon juice and process to a lumpy paste. You can alter the consistency by changing the amounts of olive oil and lemon juice, but keep the 3:1 ratio of oil to juice. (The pesto freezes well, so make several batches during the coriander season and store in small containers.)

Cook the pasta as directed on the packet and spoon over the pesto immediately so that it melts into the hot pasta. Toss well, stir in the feta cheese and sprinkle generously with grated Parmesan and freshly ground black pepper.

DISHES FOR DEBILITY

As soon as any member of the family has health problems or simply feels under-the-weather the Chinese will produce a "congee"—or *shi fan* (water rice)—to comfort and strengthen.

Congee is a Western term derived from the Anglo-Indian word for porridge, but to the Chinese these dishes are *shi fan* or water rice. Congees have been used since ancient times for a wide range of ailments. In Buddhist tradition, congee made with milk and honey was regarded as a general preventative for ill health. It was said to confer "life and beauty, ease and strength," would dispel "hunger, thirst, and Wind," as well as helping digestion and "cleansing the bladder."

The congee is basically a thin rice gruel which is made by putting one cup of rice with six cups of water in a heavy-bottomed, lidded saucepan. The pot is then simmered on the lowest possible heat on the hob for up to six hours. It needs to be stirred regularly to prevent sticking. Alternatively, you can use a slow cooker or very cool oven (such as the simmering oven on an Aga) and leave overnight—ideal if you are making congee for breakfast. Stir the mixture as soon as you can in the morning.

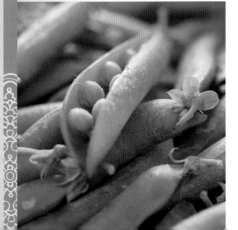

Peas and other foods can be added to congee to make a complete meal.

Plain congee is often served for breakfast in parts of China with an assortment of side dishes, such as hard-boiled eggs or steamed buns. Others prefer breakfast congee with added *hong zao* (Chinese red dates), *sheng jiang* (fresh ginger) and honey: ginger helps *qi* and Blood circulation, the red dates are calming for *shén* (Spirit) while honey helps to lubricate the digestive system and nourish the Heart—a good way to start the day.

Congee can be given a suitably therapeutic spin by adding various medicinal herbs; these are generally added mid-way through cooking. Various vegetables, meats, and spices can also be added while shrimp, chicken livers, kidneys, peas, or bamboo shoots can turn the congee into a complete therapeutic meal.

The 16th century herbalist Li Shi Zhen recommended a variety of congees in his great herbal, the *Ben Cao Gang Mu*, written between 1552 and 1578. Among his additions to a basic rice congee were:

Ginger congee: adding dried ginger to the mix to combat "Cold and Deficiency" problems that may lead to indigestion and diarrhea.

Liver congee: with chopped liver added to the mixture as a remedy for "Liver Deficiency syndromes."

Aduki bean congee: to help with fluid retention and urinary dysfunction.

Leek or onion congee: as a warming remedy for the digestive system, suitable in diarrhea.

Chestnut congee: which will tonify the Kidneys and strengthen the lower back.

Radish (*luo bo*) congee: a digestive tonic to cool the system.

Apricot seed (*xing ren*) congee: used as an expectorant for chest problems including productive coughs and asthma.

FOODS ESPECIALLY FOR WOMEN

In Chinese theory, menstruation is closely linked to the Liver, which stores Blood, while menopausal problems are seen in terms of declining Kidney energy and *jīng*. Foods that nourish and support these organs can be helpful for many women at different times of their lives.

Excessive menstruation can lead to iron-deficient anemia. In the West this tends to be treated with iron supplements while in China remedies to nourish the Blood, such as *dang gui* (Chinese angelica), are preferred. This tonic herb is traditionally cooked in stews and casseroles both for heavy periods and after childbirth as a restorative tonic. Kidney remedies like *he shou wu* (fleeceflower root) are also eaten—cooked with black beans to both restore *jīng* and nourish Blood.

Foods that can be helpful for the Liver include: celery, chicory, plums, leeks, crabs, mussels, clams, eel, liver (ox, calves', chickens', pigs', and lambs'), chives, star anise, saffron, vinegar, and wine (in moderation). Foods that can be helpful for the Kidneys include: chestnuts, grapes, Job's tear seeds, lotus (seed, fruit and root), black soybean, walnut, wheat, yam, carp, eel, chicken egg yolk, duck, kidney (calves," lambs," pigs'), mutton, pork, salt, chives, dill, cinnamon, clove, and fennel.

Chinese angelica is used to nourish the Blood and is one of the most popular women's tonic herbs.

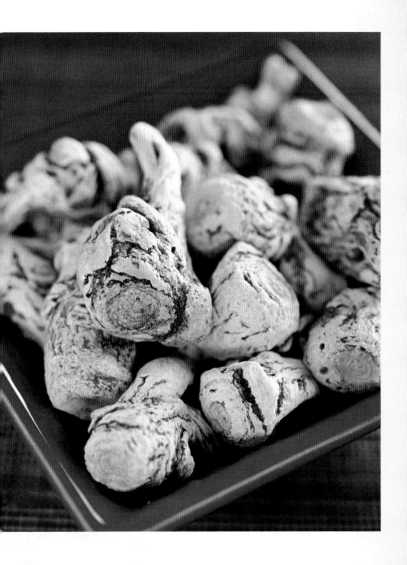

CHICKEN LIVER SOUP WITH DANG GUI AND GOU QI ZI

Serves 4

½ oz (15 g) Chinese angelica (*dang gui*)
1 oz (25 g) goji berries (*gou qi zi*)
7 oz (200 g) fresh chicken livers
1 tablespoon soy sauce
1 teaspoon sugar
1 teaspoon cornflour
freshly ground black pepper
1 tablespoon sunflower or olive oil
1 inch (2.5 cm) slice ginger root, peeled and finely chopped
1 teaspoon salt
4 pints (2.5 liters) water
1 lb (500 g) spinach
chopped coriander or parsley to garnish

This combination of livers, Chinese angelica (*dang gui*) and wolfberry fruits or goji berries (*gou qi zi*) nourishes the Liver and Blood. It is ideal for anyone with iron-deficient anemia and is also restorative in old age. Both the herbs are nourishing for *qi* and Blood and energizing for Liver and Kidneys. Spinach is cool with a sweet flavor and nourishes Blood; it is rich in minerals and is another helpful food in anemia.

Rinse the Chinese angelica and goji berries thoroughly in running water.

Combine the chicken livers with the soy sauce, sugar, cornflour, and a good grinding of pepper. In a large saucepan heat the oil and sauté the ginger and salt for about 30 seconds. Add the water, Chinese angelica and goji berries and bring to the boil, then add the chicken-liver mixture and spinach; cover with a lid and leave to simmer for 30 minutes.

To serve, sprinkle with parsley or coriander; remove the piece of Chinese angelica, but leave the goji berries to eat.

LAMB WITH DANG GUI AND GOU QI ZI

Serves 4

1 lb (500 g) lean lamb
12 shiitake mushrooms (fresh
    or dried)
2 tablespoons olive oil
3 slices ginger root, each
    about $^1/_2$ inch (1 cm) thick
2 garlic cloves, crushed
$^1/_3$ oz (10 g) Chinese angelica
    (*dang gui*)
$^1/_3$ oz (10 g) goji berries (*gou
    qi zi*)
4 pints (2.5 liters) water or
    vegetable stock
sea salt and freshly ground
    black pepper

This dish is a strengthening tonic dish for women with a tendency for anemia or menstrual irregularities, and is also ideal for anyone suffering from over-work or exhaustion. It makes a restorative meal for any condition associated with Blood Stagnation or Deficiency— the sort of health problems that may involve poor circulation or Heart irregularities.

Cut the lamb into cubes. If using dried shiitake mushrooms, soak for half an hour in warm water. Reserve the liquid to add to the stew.

Slice the soaked or fresh mushrooms. Heat the oil in a wok or large saucepan and stir-fry the lamb with the ginger for 1 minute or until lightly browned. Add the garlic, sliced mushrooms, Chinese angelica, goji berries, water or stock and salt and pepper. Cover the wok or saucepan with a lid and simmer gently for $2^1/_2$ hours.

Serve the stew with plenty of plain boiled rice or crusty bread, carrots or steamed savoy cabbage. Eat the goji berries as well, although the piece of Chinese angelica should be removed before serving.

LONGEVITY DISHES

Old age is associated with increasing *yin* and a decline in Kidney energy: factors associated with the Kidney from the five-element model—head hair, hearing, urination—can all become a problem as we age so cold, *yin* and salty foods need to be taken in moderation.

Some Chinese practitioners recommend avoiding all tropical fruits and using soy sauce instead of salt in old age. A surfeit of both fruits and salt can make the body more *yin* in nature without specifically strengthening depleted Kidney *yin* so upsetting the constitutional balance still further. Very yin foods also include crab, clams and seaweed while less *yin* foods include many fruits, ham, and shrimp. Salty foods include many shellfish, duck, ham, pork, and seaweed. Chinese tradition also recommends a daily portion of longevity tonics. Favorites include *shi hu* (orchid stems), as a daily tea to replenish jīng, and a daily sherry glass of *he shou wu* (fleeceflower) and *ren shen* (Korean ginseng) tincture.

Korean or red ginseng has been valued as a tonic herb in Europe since the 17th century.

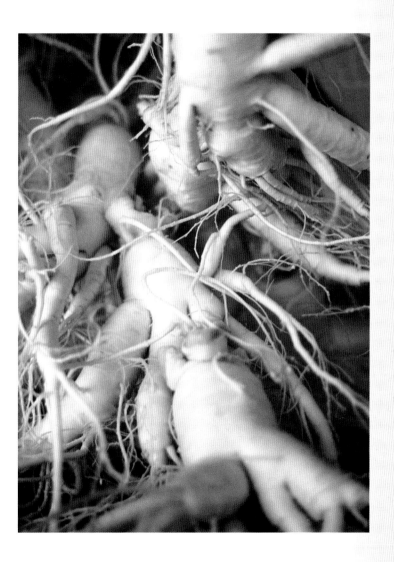

LONGEVITY PORK STEW

Serves 4–6

2 lb (1 kg) stewing pork, cut into cubes

4 tablespoons rice wine

2 tablespoons chopped coriander

2 tablespoons walnut oil

2 tablespoons brown sugar

$\frac{1}{2}$ oz (15 g) Chinese yam (*shan yao*)

$\frac{1}{2}$ oz (15 g) goji berries (*gou qi zi*)

2 pieces Korean ginseng (*ren shen*)

2 oz (50 g) shiitake mushrooms, halved or quartered

$\frac{1}{2}$ carrot, sliced

2 leeks, washed and sliced

$\frac{1}{4}$ pint (150 ml) vegetable or chicken stock

salt and pepper

This combination will tonify *qi*, nourish Kidney *yin* and tonify Blood so is an ideal dish for older people, helping to restore basic energy and *jīng*. This stew is best eaten on the second day.

Marinate the pork in the rice wine and coriander overnight or for at least four hours.

Heat the walnut oil in a large saucepan and then add the sugar. Continue heating until the sugar softens; before it starts to bubble and burn add the pork pieces. Brown the pork to seal the meat. Add the marinade, the Chinese herbs, shiitake mushrooms, carrot and leeks. Sauté gently for 2–3 minutes and then add the stock.

Cover and simmer over a low heat for about 2 hours or until the meat is tender. Add more stock if the stew becomes too dry. Before serving, cut the ginseng into bite-size pieces and if necessary, thicken the sauce with $\frac{1}{2}$ teaspoon of arrowroot or cornflour made into a paste with a little water.

Serve the stew on a bed of rice or noodles. Garnish with chopped walnuts if desired,

LAMB KIDNEYS WITH SHI HU

Serves 2

3/4 oz (20 g) dried orchid stems (*shi hu*)
1 pint (600 ml) water
4–6 lambs' kidneys, skinned, cored and quartered
1 tablespoon seasoned flour
4–6 shiitake mushrooms, quartered
1 tablespoon olive oil
2 garlic cloves, crushed
3 teaspoons cornflour
2 teaspoons paprika
1 teaspoon vegetable bouillon or a stock cube

Shi hu (orchid stem) was a favorite longevity tonic of the ancient Taoists eaten as a fresh vegetable when in season. The herb is also said to increase sexual vigor and combat fatigue associated with excessive sexual activity. As a potent Kidney tonic, shi hu also relieves lower back and knee pains and restores Body Fluids. The spices used here are warming and invigorating.

Chop the dried orchid stems and cover with the water. Bring to the boil, cover the pan and simmer for 10–15 minutes. Leave to cool.

Coat the prepared kidney quarters in seasoned flour and then sauté both the kidneys and shiitake mushrooms, separately, in the olive oil in a wok for about 5 minutes or until thoroughly cooked. Remove from the pan and put to one side. Add the garlic to the pan juices and sauté for a few seconds mixing well; then sprinkle the cornflour and paprika into the pan and continue stirring over a low heat.

Remove and discard the orchid stems from its boiling liquid, add the vegetable bouillon (or stock cube) and then pour this into the wok. Bring to a boil and simmer to thicken. Add the kidneys and shiitake to the wok and simmer gently to reheat, adjust the seasoning and serve with boiled rice.

TEA

Drinking tea (*cha*) in China reputedly goes back to the days of Shen Nong (see page 10), who discovered the drink when some leaves from the tea plant (*Camellia sinensis*) accidentally fell into a cauldron of water that was boiling nearby and he found the result was a delicious and restorative drink.

Tea drinking is very much part of everyday life in China: railway stations, airports, in fact anywhere where people are likely to wait, are traditionally equipped with a large hot water boiler. People carry with them a screw-top jar containing their tea leaves and these can simply be topped up from any convenient hot water boiler.

Traditionally, tea is said to have a bitter-sweet taste and is dry. Differently processed teas also have different characters. Green tea and oolong tea are classified as cooling. In contrast, black tea, the traditional

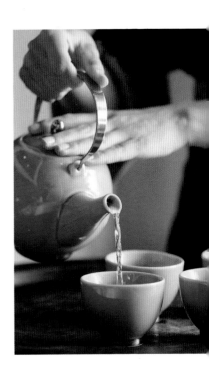

Numerous varieties of tea are drunk in China, many with therapeutic properties.

fermented variety widely drunk in Europe, India, and North America, is warming.

Modern research has also highlighted different properties:

Green teas: These are rich in fluoride and can be used to combat tooth decay. They are also antioxidant and have been shown to combat both stomach and skin cancers and boost the immune system.

Oolong teas: These are effective as digestive remedies and are diuretic; Japanese research suggests that some oolong tea can reduce high blood pressure and limit the risk of atherosclerosis.

Black tea: This contains stimulating alkaloids that can give a temporary boost to the nervous system and dispel tiredness. Black tea without milk is a traditional Chinese remedy both for diarrhea and hangovers.

In China green and oolong teas tend to be drunk on hot days as a cooling remedy while black tea is preferred in cold winter. Among the many therapeutic Chinese teas are:

Gunpowder or *zhu cha* (pearl tea): A large-leaf green tea that is especially rich in fluoride: two cups contain the body's entire daily requirement of fluoride (2 mg).

Liu xi (flowing stream): A green tea that is traditionally drunk for digestive disorders and constipation; it is said to help relieve any discomfort after a heavy meal.

Bai hao yinzhen (white down silver needles): A white tea from Fujian province, it is used to reduce Heat, combat Dampness and stimulate the intestines.

Pu erh: An oolong tea from Yunnan province generally sold in compressed bricks, balls, or bowl shapes; it is highly regarded as a digestive remedy and is now known to reduce blood cholesterol levels after a fatty meal. A strong cup of *pu erh* tea is a traditional hangover cure.

THERAPEUTIC DRINKS

Tonic wines are a long-established way of taking therapeutic herbs. Many use a single herb, although various combinations aimed at specific organs and energy problems have been developed over the centuries. These herbal wines can also be added, like brandy or vermouth, in cooking to provide flavor and health benefits.

Alcohol has been used to extract the active constituents of medicinal plants for at least 2,000 years in both Eastern and Western traditions. The alcohol acts as a preservative and if the resulting tinctures are stored in a cool dark place they will generally retain their health-giving properties for up to two years. In China rice wine (*huang jiu*) is generally used. *Huang jiu* itself regarded as a tonic in pregnancy and breastfeeding.

A stronger mixture can be made by using spirits—traditionally Chinese white spirit (*bai jiu*) although vodka makes a suitable substitute. Brandy is also usable although gin should be avoided as it contains juniper berries which have their own, possibly unwanted, therapeutic properties.

MAKING TONIC WINES

The simplest method is to put the herbs and alcohol—usually in the proportion 1:5 weight to volume of herbs to alcohol—4 oz of herb to 1 pint alcohol (100 g of herb to 500 ml alcohol)—in a glass jar and store in a cool dark place for a month, shaking the jar occasionally. The resulting tincture can then be strained or pressed from the herb and stored in a clean bottle, and the herb is generally discarded. For tonic wines the usual dosage is a sherry glass daily; if stronger alcohol is used then 1–2 teaspoons diluted with a little water is usual.

HERBAL TONIC WINES TO MAKE AT HOME

Huang qi jiu (milk vetch): Usually made from slices of dried root and rice wine, this is used to tonify *yang qi* and *wèi qi*. It is especially useful for those suffering from any weakness in the limbs, shortness of breath, or palpitations and sweating associated with *qi* Deficiency.

Hong zao jiu (red dates): Made from whole red Chinese dates, this is used to replenish Spleen and Stomach *qi* and nourish Blood. It is a good one to make with brandy and use as an after-dinner drink to help digest heavy meals. Instead of discarding the dates, chop them finely and add to fruit salads, meat dishes, or fruit cakes.

Dang gui jiu (Chinese angelica): Best made from sliced angelica

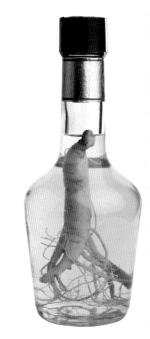

Commercially-made tonic wines and liqueurs sometimes contain herbs.

rather than a whole root, with brandy, this is a traditional woman's tonic to nourish Blood and invigorate the circulation. A tablespoon in water will help to relieve period pain. After childbirth it is often combined with *bai shao yao* (white peony), *wu wei zi* (schizandra fruits), *shan yao* (Chinese yam), *du zhong* (eucommia bark), *gan cao* (liquorice), and *gou qi zi* (wolfberry fruits). Use equal amounts of the Dang gui and the first three herbs to half as much of the last three.

Xi yang shen jiu (American ginseng): Made from slices of dried root, this helps to strengthen *qi*, nourish *yin*, generate fluids and also helps recovery from feverish illnesses or for throat problems and coughs. It is

Chinese red dates are used in various tonic wines.

pleasant as an aperitif or can be used to marinate duck or chicken.

Hu tao ren jiu (walnut wine): Made from shelled nuts, this is used as a tonic for Lungs and Kidneys and to nourish *jīng*; it is useful for back pain related to Kidney Deficiency and for respiratory problems. Best made from vodka, it is also a useful flavoring for fruit salads and can be added to meat marinades.

Dang shen (bellflower): Made from chopped root, this is used as a general *qi* tonic and to stimulate Blood production. It is particularly good for Spleen, Stomach, and Lung and significantly less expensive than *ren shen* (Korean ginseng).

Gou qi zi jiu (goji berries): Made from the whole berries and rice wine, this is used as a tonic for Liver and Kidney *yin* and to improve the eyesight. *Gou qi zi jiu* is a sweet-tasting wine that can also be used to flavor fruit salads and added to sauces. **Caution**: Be sure to buy good-quality herbs—cases of *gou qi zi* contaminated with ephedrine have been recorded.

Shan zha hong zao jui (hawthorn berries and red dates): Chinese hawthorn berries are larger than the European variety and both these and red dates should be chopped before use in this recipe, with a pinch of cinnamon and a tablespoon of brown

sugar added to the mixture. This wine promotes digestion, disperses Food Stagnation and eases abdominal bloating. It is ideal as a dressing for fruit salads to make a therapeutic dessert following a large meal.

Ren shen huang qi jiu (Korean ginseng and milk vetch): Use twice as much *huang qi* as *ren shen* to give a strong *qi* tonic; especially useful for Lung weakness or following influenza. While the *huang qi* should be discarded after use, *ren shen* can be salvaged, chopped and added to energizing meat stews and casseroles.

Shan yao jiu (Chinese yam): Made from slices of yam root rather than whole pieces, this is used as a tonic for Spleen and Stomach to improve digestion and also to strengthen Kidney and Liver *qi* and *jīng*.

Du zhong jui (eucommia bark): Made from chopped pieces of bark, this is used to tonify Kidney and Liver *qi* and *jīng*; also helpful for back pain associated with Kidney Deficiency and in infertility or impotence.

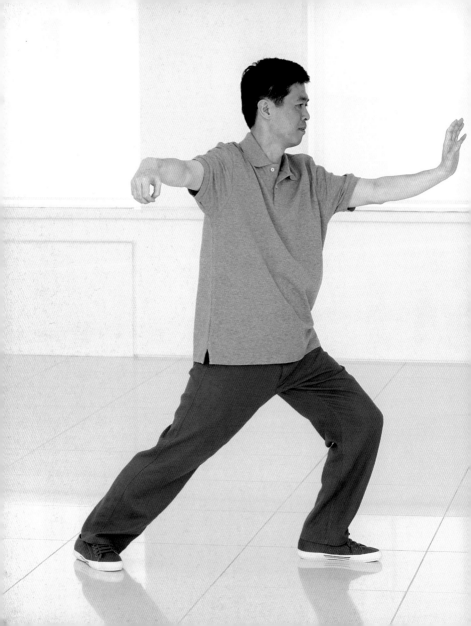

Part 6

BODY WORK

CHINESE EXERCISE THERAPIES

Chinese exercise therapies are included as one of the "eight limbs" of healing—meditation, diet, astrology, geomancy, massage, herbalism, and acupuncture being the others. They are also closely linked to martial arts, which involve mobilizing the *qi* in order to defeat one's opponents.

While Chinese medicine talks of the various forms of *qi* that circulate in the body and can be equated with vital energy or an inner life force, the concept can seem somewhat nebulous to Westerners. Feeling one's *qi* brings this life force sharply into focus as something that is present and tangible

Qigong is China's oldest form of exercise therapy dating to the days of the Yellow Emperor and the Taoists, and developed over the centuries by Buddhist monks, traditional Chinese doctors and martial arts practitioners. Traditionally, it is believed to

eliminate disease and prolong life, using exercises that strengthen and focus the *qi*. Experienced practitioners are able not only to use *qigong* to strengthen their own *qi* but to then use their *qi* to heal others in *qigong* massage without depleting their own store of energy.

Although *qi* is generally translated as "vital energy" it also means breath while *gong* can mean both the time spent acquiring a skill, the quality of the practice, and the actual attainment of the art—so *qigong* may be translated both as breathing exercise or energy skill. "Breathing exercise" seems reminiscent of yoga

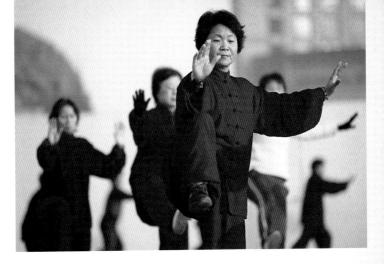

but the healing aspects of *qigong* in massage makes it into a powerful therapeutic technique.

Qigong is also a valuable self-help technique to strengthen our own *qi* in order to combat disease and improve health and well-being. Although it is comparatively easy to feel one's *qi*, using any exercise therapy takes practice.

Groups exercising in the open air can be seen in many Chinese cities.

T'AI-CHI

T'ai-chi—sometimes called *t'ai-chi chu'an*—is one of the many styles of *qigong* and is probably better known in the West. It is often taught as a martial art, but it also has a spiritual dimension. *T'ai* means great while *chi* here is an alternate spelling for *ji* (not *qi*) and means ultimate, so *t'ai chi* means great ultimate; *ch'uan* translates as fist so *t'ai-chi ch'uan* is usually translated as boundless fist or great extremes boxing.

"Supreme ultimate" (*taiji*) is a concept that occurs in both Taoism and Confucian philosophy and represents the fusion of *yin* and *yang* symbolized by the familiar *taijitu* symbol.

QIGONG EXERCISES

Qigong exercises are generally divided into three main groups—passive, active, and a combination of the two.

The first of these is a passive, static type of exercise, which involves focusing on *qi*, *shén* (spirit) or *yi* (mind) and is sometimes described as "training the mind." The more active form focuses on breathing routines and is known as dynamic *qigong*; while the third, a combination of both, is probably the form most familiar in the West and includes various postures and movements for training the body.

Passive and active *qigong* can be seen as *yin* and *yang* respectively: *yin* is passive and meditative—"training the mind," while *yang* is active and moving—"training the breath." Put them together to create a whole and you have dynamic-

quiescent postures and movements where every action is controlled, conscious and complete: the combined *taiju* model as in *t'ai-chi ch'uan*.

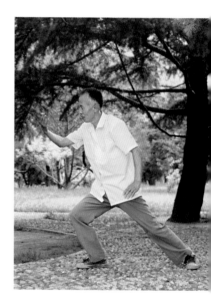

Elderly Chinese practicing *qigong* in public parks is a common sight in parts of China.

FEELING *QI*

1 *Qigong* is all about feeling and strengthening *qi* and the easiest way to do this is simply to stand with feet shoulder-width apart in the quiescent *qi* pose (see page 338). Relax with the arms loosely by your side and clear the mind of thoughts.

2 *Qi* starts to pool in the hands, which begin to feel warm and tingling. Breath deeply into the lower abdomen to help relaxation. After a few minutes slowly raise the hands in front of you, palms facing in, until they are about 12 inches (30 cm) apart. As you breath in move the hands closer together but not touching, and as you breath out move them away again.

3 The sensation of heat in the hands seems to develop a magnetic force of its own—a tangible energy that has its own resistance and elasticity. This is the *qi* that in *t'ai-chi ch'uan* can be hurled at opponents or in *qigong* massage used to re-energize damaged tissues.

4 Having "pooled the *qi*" do not waste it: use the power in your hands to massage any area of the body that is

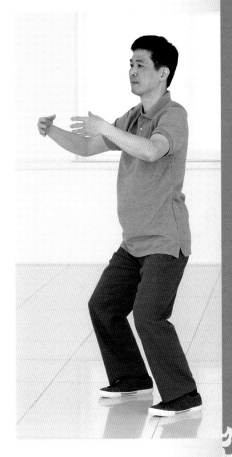

feeling weak, or else simply restore it to your Kidneys by placing the hands, firmly, palms downward in the small of the back.

QIGONG BREATHING

Breath control is a core aspect of dynamic *qigong* and involves movement, not just breathing routines. The act of breathing is commonly divided into chest breathing and abdominal breathing.

CHEST BREATHING

In chest breathing the middle *dan tien* is said to be energized. The *dan tien*—literally the "elixir field" and often called the "sea of *qi* " in the West—is the area about three fingers' widths below the navel and two fingers' widths behind the surface, which is one of the major areas of the body where *qi* is stored. This area is sometimes called the lower *dan tien*, with the upper *dan tien* corresponding to the "third eye" at a point between the eyebrows, while the middle *dan tien* corresponds with the Heart. Here the chest expands as you inhale and relaxes as you exhale. Practice involves taking regular breaths, purely expanding and relaxing the chest without moving the abdomen.

ABDOMINAL BREATHING

In abdominal breathing the abdomen moves in and out as you breathe. It is best to start by placing your hands on the lower abdomen, level with the navel and feel it rise and fall with each breath in and out. Once you have perfected this sort of breathing, the hands can be held, palms facing, in front of the navel to help focus *qi* on the lower *dan tien*.

BREATHING EXERCISES

Both these forms of breathing should be practiced regularly, starting with two-minute sessions for each and gradually building up to five minutes of steady deep chest or abdominal breathing. Both can be practiced either sitting down or standing up. All these breathing routines can be practiced on a daily basis: they do not require complex preparations—sitting comfortably and quietly at an office desk without interruption is just as suitable as practicing cross-legged on a remote hillside.

Breathing exercises are often seen as an aspect of meditation, clearing the mind, focusing on the breath, and becoming one with the universe. Meditation is taught in many different ways, with students often encouraged to focus on a complex mandala or chant a specific mantra. Others suggest a simple half smile: all one need do is lift the corners of the mouth slightly in a half smile and hold the expression for the space of three breaths. Repeat six times or more each day.

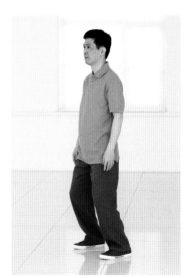

WU CHI

1 *Wu chi*, supreme emptiness, is a focused breathing routine practiced only when standing. Legs should be at shoulder-width with feet facing forward and arms loosely hanging at the sides. The knees should be relaxed, slightly bent and not locked straight, and the posture as upright as possible not bending forward or leaning back.

2 As you breathe in, feel the energy of the breath slowly travelling down to the lower *dan tien*. Continue with the posture and breathing exercises for as long as it feels comfortable.

PASSIVE QIGONG

Typical of the passive exercises is a very simple standing pose *zhan zhuang* or "standing like a tree," which is designed to calm the Heart and so achieve a peaceful mind. Simple standing is far from simple and involves a total of 18 separate and conscious movements:

STANDING LIKE A TREE

1 The feet should be flat on the ground, shoulder-wide apart with the weight evenly distributed.

2 The knees must be relaxed and slightly bent so that *qi* and Blood can flow freely.

3 The hip joints need to be relaxed.

4 The crotch needs to be slightly tensed to avoid any leakage of *qi* from the "lower door." This is usually achieved by lifting the knee caps to give a lightness to the lower limbs and then lifting the perineum slightly.

5 The anus is similarly tensed and lifted in the same way.

6 Next the stomach needs to be pulled in above the pubic bone, which helps to restrain the primordial qi and improve *qi* flow through the body.

7 The waist must be relaxed to allow the *qi* to sink back to the *dan tien*. Relaxing the waist is usually achieved by lifting the shoulders and then relaxing them downward immediately while breathing out.

8 The chest must then be pulled in to expand the thoracic cavity.

9 Next the back should be stretched so that the vertebrae are upright and the shoulders droop evenly.

10 Drooping the shoulder joints also helps the neck to relax.

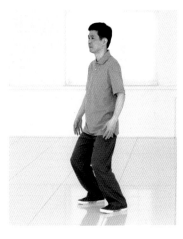

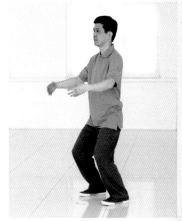

11 The elbows are next—they need to be bent slightly and then dropped.

12 The elbows then need to be moved gently away from the body so that the armpits are open and hollow.

13 The wrists should be relaxed so that *qi* can flow through to the fingers—this is achieved by gently hollowing the palm and bending the fingers.

14 Next suspend the head by imagining it hanging from a thread so that it is upright and central to the body.

15 Tuck in the chin.

16 Close the eyes; not tightly shut but with eyelids drooping.

17 The lips and teeth need to be gently closed so that the molars are in the biting position.

18 Move the tongue so that it is touching the upper palate.

Having achieved this far-from-simple standing pose, breathe calmly, clear the mind and concentrate on the *dan tien* area. Skilled *qigong* exponents will often stand in this way for several hours focusing on their *qi*—try it for 5 minutes to start with and sit down immediately if you start to feel faint.

DYNAMIC QIGONG

Dynamic *qigong* combines breathing with simple movement to encourage better breath control. By breathing in more and out less *qigong* exponents believe they can strengthen inner energies: practice is enhanced by simple movements.

THE HEALTHY WALK

One of the easiest exercises is called the healthy walk and starts from the standing pose of quiescent *qigong*.

1 Walk forward with the heel touching the ground and the toes lifted high, while relaxing the head and waist.

2 Swing the arms gently from side to side so that one hand comes to rest on the *dan tien* at the completion of each step.

3 Look from left and right while walking as if admiring flowers.

4 Breathing should be through the nose—breathing in for two steps and out for one, using chest breathing for a few steps and then abdominal breathing. **NB**: If suffering from heart disease or high blood pressure breathe naturally instead.

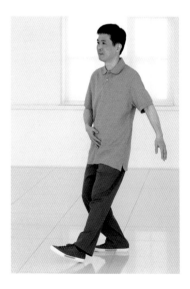

THE ENERGETIC HEALTHY WALK

Qigong experts teach various forms of the healthy walk: some encourage more vigorous arm movements, swinging the arms up to head height and twisting the body at the same time to look at the hand.

1 Start from the basic standing position and take a step forward with your left foot, heel first to the ground as before, at the same time swing the right arm upward so the hand is at head height and the elbow slightly bent while breathing in.

2 Gradually swing the left arm upward while breathing out, the right arm back, while placing the left foot firmly on the ground and raise the right heel.

3 Move the right leg forward, heel to ground first as before while breathing in with, by now, the left arm at head height and the right arm swinging slightly backward.

4 Repeat the earlier heel to toe movement and breathing sequence, while moving the left arm down and the right arm preparing to move upward, taking you back to the first step and the left foot moving forward.

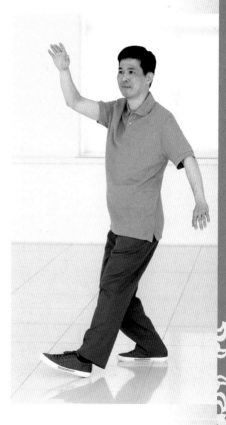

QIGONG SEQUENCES

Having mastered passive *qigong*, breathing and simple movements, the next stage is to put all these elements together into a structured sequence combining both passive mediation and active breathing. There are many *qigong* movement sequences designed to invigorate and strengthen different parts of the body or to combat inherent weaknesses.

Routines range from the simple to some that approach lengthy *t'ai-chi* cycles in complexity but most have a clear health focus. The *baduanjin* or "eight silk brocade" exercises consists of a series of quite simple movements—only three or four to each stage—that progressively relax the muscles, stretch the limbs and chest, improve the circulation, strengthen the digestive system, nervous system, spine and back, ending with routines to energize the entire body and help concentration.

Other cycles are more lengthy: *dayan qigong* or "wild goose" *qigong* consists of a total of 128 movements that imitate the motion of the wild goose. The first 64 are designed to help postnatal *qi* while the second half is for prenatal *qi*. The cycle originated with the Taoists and, like much Taoist therapy, is believed to delay ageing and prolong life.

All *qigong* routines involve an opening sequence—activating and moving *qi*—and then a closing cycle that will return the invigorated *qi* to its storage areas. If the exercise is not completed then the *qi* is not returned to storage and vital energy can be lost so that the entire effort will have been wasted.

Qigong is often performed in the open air emphasizing the importance of breath.

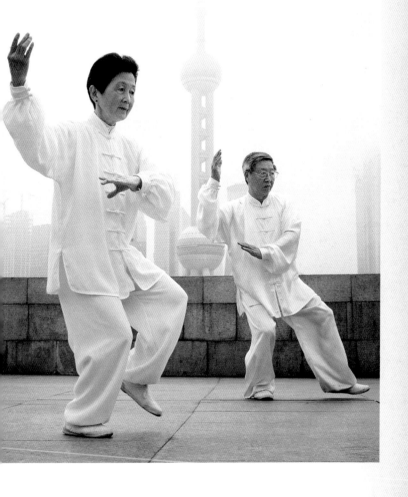

STANDING EIGHT PIECES OF BROCADE

HOLDING THE PALMS TO HEAVEN

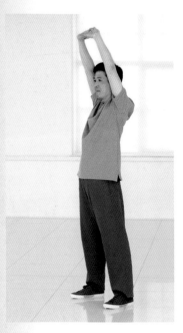 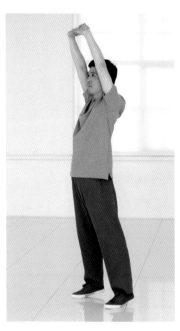

1 Stand with your feet shoulder-width apart and with hands at your side. Close your eyes and calm the mind while breathing regularly. Once the mind is calm, open your eyes, interlock your fingers and raise the arms above your head without bending the arms.

2 At the same time raise your heels from the ground in the "double hands hold up the heavens" pose. At the same time you should try to focus your *qi* on the lower *dan tien*.

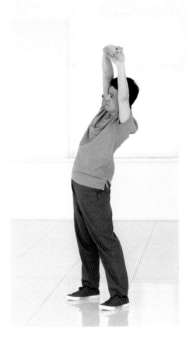

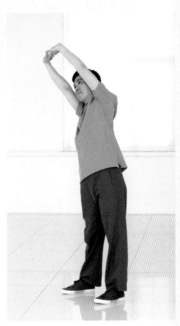

3 Drop the heels to the ground and sway to the left with the hands still interlocked and the arms still above the head.

4 Then sway to the right. The hands should then be lowered to the front of the body. This sequence is repeated 24 times.

DRAWING THE BOW TO SHOOT THE EAGLE

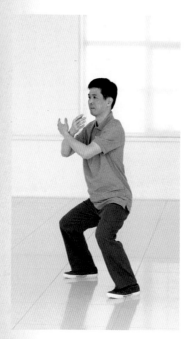

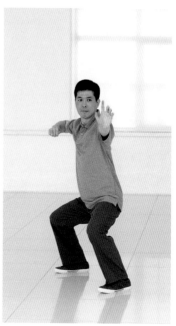

5 Step to the right with the right leg and squat down as if riding a horse. Relax the hands and then lift them to the chest, holding them with the wrists crossed.

6 Separate the hands, extending the left hand to the side and moving the right to be above the right breast, as though pulling the string of a bow. The eyes should be focused on a distant point.

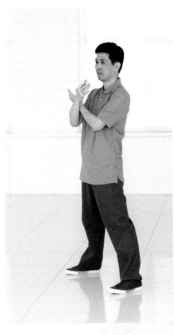

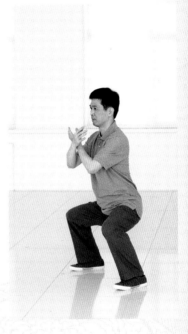

7 Stand up straight, lower the hands, circle them up toward the chest and cross them.

8 Repeat the sequence: start by squatting with wrists crossed.

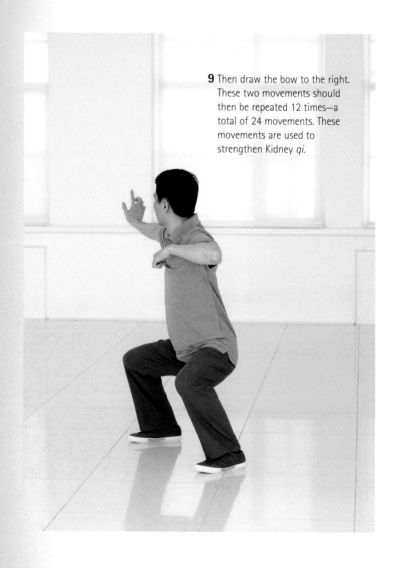

9 Then draw the bow to the right. These two movements should then be repeated 12 times—a total of 24 movements. These movements are used to strengthen Kidney *qi*.

SEPARATING HEAVEN AND EARTH

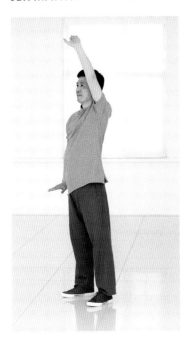 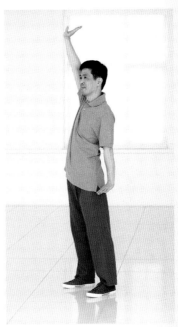

10 Stand once more so that the legs are shoulder-width apart then move both hands to the front of the stomach with the palms facing upward. Raise the left hand above your head, pushing upward, and at the same time lower the right palm to your side pushing downward.

11 Change your arms and repeat the pushing. Repeat this cycle 12 times—a total of 24 movements.

THE WISE OWL GAZES BACKWARD

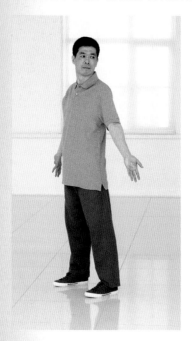
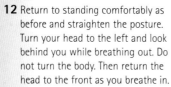
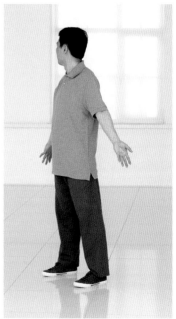

12 Return to standing comfortably as before and straighten the posture. Turn your head to the left and look behind you while breathing out. Do not turn the body. Then return the head to the front as you breathe in.

13 Turn to the right and exhale, looking behind you and then return to the front while breathing in as before. Repeat this 12 times in either direction, a total of 24 movements. This movement is said to heal "five weaknesses and seven injuries"— meaning the five *yin zang* organs and the seven emotions.

THE BIG BEAR TURNS FROM SIDE TO SIDE

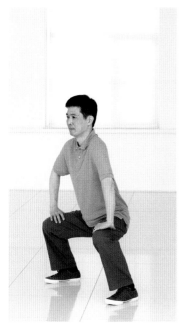

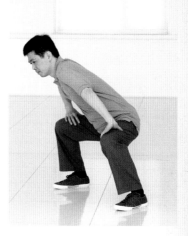

14 The next movement is to prevent any build-up of Heart Fire. From the basic standing pose, step with the right leg to the right, while still facing forward and squat as if riding a horse as before. Place your hands on top of your knees with the thumbs on the outer side of the thighs.

15 Press down heavily on the left leg and rotate the torso from the hips, leaning first to the right side and forward, looking slightly to the left.

16 Then as you sweep your torso in an arc forward and to the left, transfer your weight to the left leg and turn your head to look slightly to the right. Turn 12 times either way giving 24 movements in all.

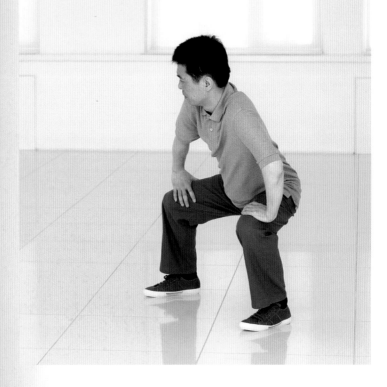

TOUCH THE SKY, PRESS THE EARTH

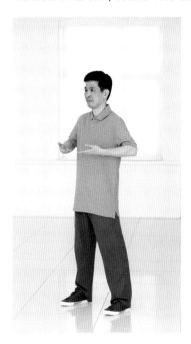

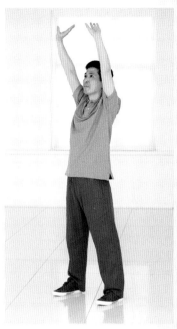

17 Return to the standing position. This movement is designed to strengthen Kidney *qi*, relieve any Kidney *qi* stagnation which may damage *jīng*, and also boost *wèi qi*. Press the palms downward, then move them to the chest with the palms facing upward.

18 Twist the hands out and away from you as you continue to lift your arms above your head with the palms facing upward. Focus the mind on the *ming men* (life gate) acu-point (GV4) which is on the spine at the second lumbar vertebra.

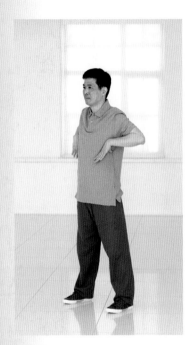 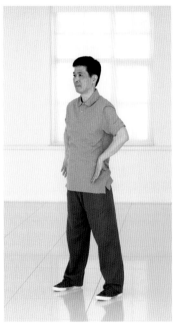

19 Stay like this for three seconds, then lower your hands to your chest with your fingers pointing downward and to the front of your body and your thumbs pointing downward and to the back of your body.

20 Continue lowering your hands to the hips.

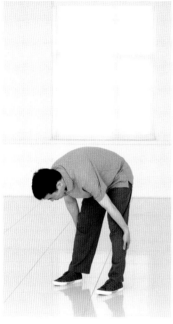

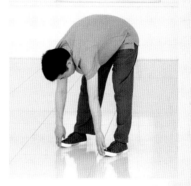

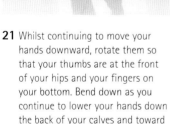

21 Whilst continuing to move your hands downward, rotate them so that your thumbs are at the front of your hips and your fingers on your bottom. Bend down as you continue to lower your hands down the back of your calves and toward your ankles.

22 Finally, run your hands along the sides of your feet and hold your toes, pulling up slightly to tense the whole body and focusing the mind back on the *yong quan* acu-point (bubbling spring) KI1. Stay in this pose for three seconds before returning to the original standing pose. Repeat this 16 times.

PUNCHING WITH ANGRY EYES

23 This movement is said to strengthen *qi* flow and muscle strength. During the movement it is important to focus the mind on the total activity: imagine you really are punching someone and your *qi* will move out along the arm to enhance the movement. In this sequence start by taking up the squatting position as if riding a horse, as in step 5, Drawing the bow to shoot the eagle (see page 346), only this time hold the body erect with the hands made into fists beside the waist.

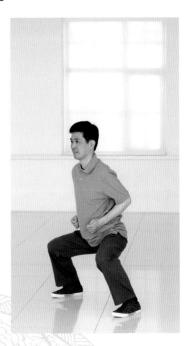

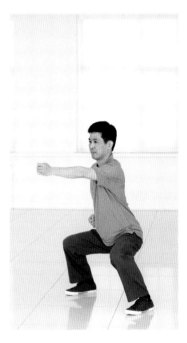 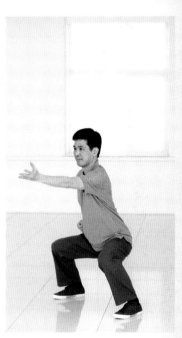

24 Tighten both fists then extend the left arm forward in a twisting, punching motion.

25 End the punch by opening the palm and twisting the hand, bringing it back to the original stance. Tighten both hands again and repeat turning to the right, first punching and then opening the palm. Repeat this 8 times to each side, a total of 16 times.

RAISING THE HEELS

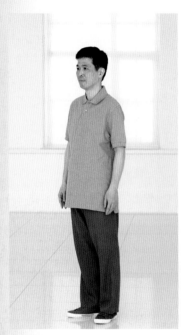

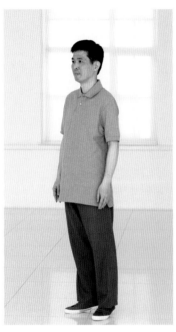

26 This closing sequence helps to restore and retain the *qi* and rebalance energies. The final movement in the *baduanjin* sequence involves starting from the original standing pose, with both hands hanging naturally at the side.

27 Keep the mind calm and then push yourself onto your toes as high as you can before lowering the feet to the floor with a rocking motion. Repeat this 24 times.

28 When you have finished resume the simple standing position and breath smoothly and regularly for three minutes.

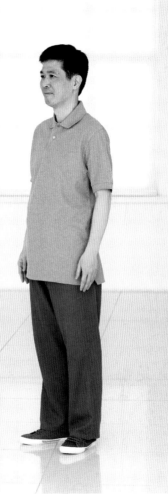

QIGONG MASSAGE

Qigong massage is sometimes described as a combination of traditional Chinese massage, Chinese pointing therapy and acupressure—applying the pointing and tapping techniques to acu-points but with the healer using *qi* transmission to apply their own *qi* to energize the treated areas.

A clearly focused mind able to move *qi* and channel energy is essential, so—in Taoist belief—is oneness with the universe, the source of all *qi*. *Tui na* or Chinese massage techniques are traditionally divided into eight *yang* and *yin* applications. *Yang* techniques are "pushing and swaying," scattering, comforting, and "pounding and knocking" while gentler *yin* methods involve "linking-dredging," reinforcing *qi*, "kneading and pinching," and "reconciling collaterals."

DEFINING THE TERMS

The labels are far from self-explanatory with pushing and swaying, for example, involving repeated sequences of pressing down on the patient with both fists, clutching and squeezing the flesh or stroking the area being treated. Linking and dredging involves gently sweeping the fingers over the area being treated, using a scrubbing motion, smoothing the area and then pulling gently on joints. In the reinforcing *qi* technique, masseurs concentrate their own *qi* in their palms to generate heat and then press, vibrate or quiver their palms across the affected area.

Yang massage techniques are used for strains, trauma, pain, and swelling in tendons and muscles, Blood Stagnation, insomnia,

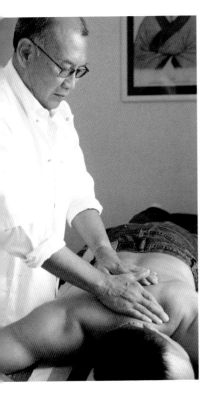

In *qigong* massage masters are able to mobilize their *qi* to help patients.

Treatments are applied not just to affected areas but to the relevant acu-points and channels. As the *Nei Jing* (see page 10) has it: "No matter how the child is given birth to, how the disease is produced, how the patient is cured, how the illness is started, how the study is begun, how the work is ended, all are based on the twelve channels, so the learning it roughly is easy, but mastering it precisely is difficult."

Traditional Chinese hospitals generally have a *qigong* department where experienced masters teach basic *qigong* techniques to patients to help combat chronic diseases such as cancer, as well as harnessing their own *qi* in massage treatments for the severely ill. By concentrating their energy into their hands experienced *qigong* masseurs can stimulate the paralyzed limbs of stroke patients or encourage movement in brain-damaged babies.

numbness, and paralysis, while *yin* techniques are applied for *qi* and Blood Deficiency syndromes, physical weakness, paralysis associated with Cold and Damp, swellings, limb injuries, obstructions to the Channels and post-injury weaknesses.

ALL ABOUT T'AI-CHI

Like *qigong*, *t'ai-chi* (or *taiji*) has developed as an exercise therapy for controlling *qi* and improving health that has been practiced for centuries. Unlike *qigong*, however, it is usually classified as a martial art and can involve a form of boxing.

T'ai-chi has steadily gained popularity since the early 1900s, when teachers began to introduce the routines to the West. *T'ai-chi* practice generally includes an emphasis on healthy lifestyle and good physical fitness, meditation to calm the mind and focus *qi*, and a martial arts aspect with the emphasis on self-defence.

Five distinct traditional schools or styles have developed over the years, each named after individuals and families that reputedly originated and perpetuated each method:

● Chen style founded by Chen Wangting (1580–1660)
● Yang style after Yang Lu-ch'an (1799–1872)
● Wu or Wu-Hao style developed by Wu Yuxiang (1813–1880)
● Wu Family style developed by Wu Ch'uan-yu (1834–1902)
● Sun style founded by Sun Lu-t'ang (1861–1932)

The most commonly taught method in the West are the Yang and Wu Family styles.

NEW DEVELOPMENTS

These traditional styles have been augmented with an assortment of routines that have developed over the past few years, some incorporating or merging parts of the traditional sequences. One of the better known is the Lee style, reputedly derived from movements created by Ho Hsieh Lee around 1000 BCE that were passed through the Lee family until the 1930s, when these were taught to Chee Soo, who then actively promoted the style in the West and also combined it with *qigong* techniques. The various styles can be extremely long and complex: the Wu style has 108 movements, the long Yang form has 103, the Sun style 98 and the Lee style up to 185.

MEMORIZING THE SEQUENCES

T'ai-chi training starts with memorizing these sequences of dynamic poses that combine abdominal breathing, and hand and leg movements. Once this solo form is perfected, students move on to combative exercises that may be conducted empty-handed or involve some form of weapon such as wooden sticks or swords. Most students who study *t'ai chi* stay with the solo form using it purely as an exercise therapy. In China large groups of people regularly practice

t'ai chi in the open air each morning, either working individually or in a more organized class.

Its practice is said to improve balance, flexibility and cardiovascular fitness in the elderly and is particularly encouraged among sufferers from multiple sclerosis and Parkinson's disease. It is also promoted as a means of relieving stress and anxiety and encouraging relaxation and general health improvements.

A key benefit of *t'ai-chi*, argue some exponents, is that it can strengthen *jīng*—fundamental essence. *Jīng* is equated here with an inner strength that is not the same as excessive physical strength or with an inherently strong physique. It is argued that constant *t'ai-chi* practice can help to build this inner strength so that in martial arts it can be harnessed to overcome opponents. *Jīng* and *qi* together are mobilized in t'ai chi and spread throughout the body so that the energy is there—like water kept under pressure—to be released as required.

T'AI-CHI PRELIMINARY EXERCISES

T'ai-chi exercise routines can be long and complex but they are often performed by adepts quite quickly, rather like an elegant and fluid dance, so with practice, the entire sequence can take 15–30 minutes.

It is important to start slowly and focus on each movement as well as the breath, and practice until it becomes almost second nature. Each extended *t'ai-chi* sequence is developed from individual movements, each with distinctive names. Some names describe the actual movement while others suggest imaginary activities or the figure's appearance. The individual movements can be regarded as preliminary exercises that should be learned and practiced until gradually the whole sequence becomes instinctive.

The full style is broken down into shorter stretches that makes it easier

to learn and these short sequences can be practiced on their own as a single routine, with a closing movement at the end to return the *qi* to its proper place.

Many of the individual movements are repeated several times during a full routine and make useful starting points for practice. As with *qigong*, *t'ai-chi* exercises generally start with a simple standing posture to focus the mind and calm the breath ready for exercise.

Learning complex *t'ai chi* sequences requires regular practice, usually starting with basic exercises.

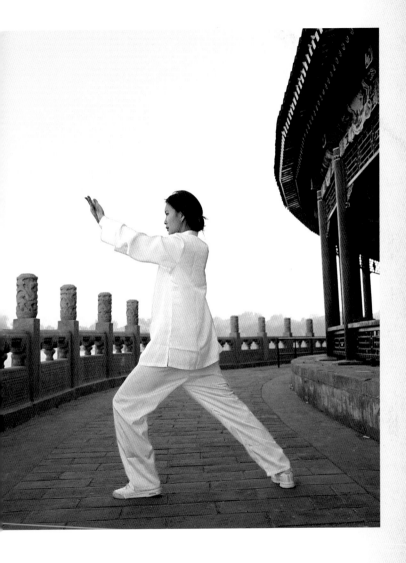

OPENING POSTURE (*QI SHI*)

This sequence helps to relax the neck and shoulders and ease tension in the arms and hands.

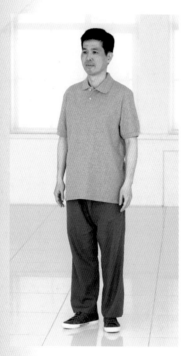 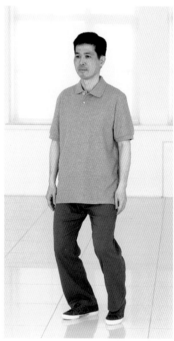

1 Stand calmly and relaxed in an upright position with the feet close together but not touching. This is the phase of *wu chi* (empty state), see page 337.

2 Bend the knees slightly so you are in *zhan zhuang* (standing like a tree), see page 338. Breathe easily and comfortably.

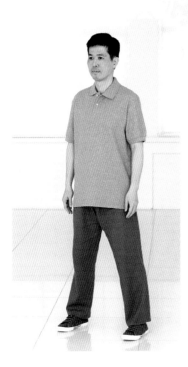

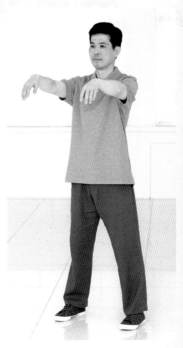

3 Then on an outward breath, slide the left foot further to the left so that the feet are shoulder-width apart with the toes pointing forward and the weight evenly distributed.

4 Gently raise both arms up, palms and fingers facing down, to about shoulder height, whilst straightening the knees.

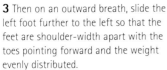

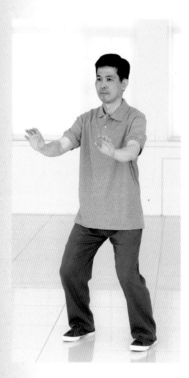

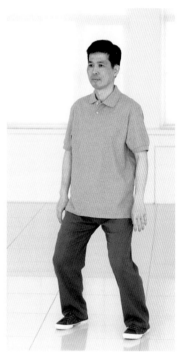

5 Breathe naturally and on an outward breath drop both the arms, palms down and fingers up, to *dan tien* height, lowering the knees once more.

6 Finally, lower both hands back to the sides.

LEFT GRASPING THE SPARROW'S TAIL (*LAN QUE WEI ZOU*)

WARD OFF (*PENG*)

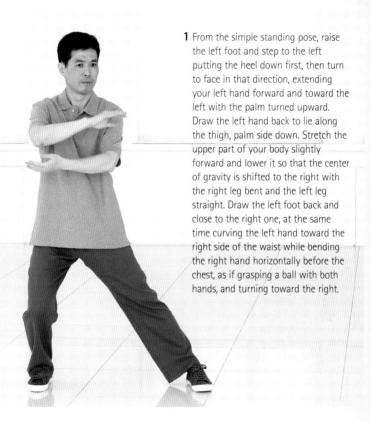

1 From the simple standing pose, raise the left foot and step to the left putting the heel down first, then turn to face in that direction, extending your left hand forward and toward the left with the palm turned upward. Draw the left hand back to lie along the thigh, palm side down. Stretch the upper part of your body slightly forward and lower it so that the center of gravity is shifted to the right with the right leg bent and the left leg straight. Draw the left foot back and close to the right one, at the same time curving the left hand toward the right side of the waist while bending the right hand horizontally before the chest, as if grasping a ball with both hands, and turning toward the right.

ROLL BACK (*LU*)

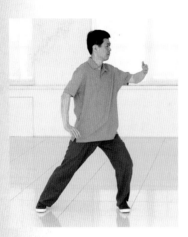 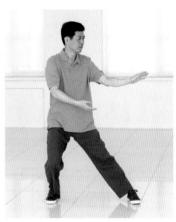

2 Next lift the left hand outward, bent toward the left as if to ward off a blow to the level of the shoulders. At the same time swing the right hand downward to the right, while breathing out, and place it beside the right thigh and stretch the left foot out and lean forward. The eyes should look at the left forearm. This is "ward off left" (*peng zuo*).

3 The next stage is to inhale while stretching the left hand forward, turning the palm downward while turning the right palm upward and stretching it forward until below the left wrist. This is "roll back" (*lu*).

PRESS (*JI*)

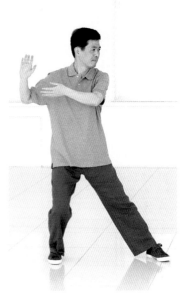

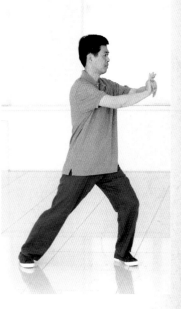

4 Move the hands downward past the abdomen and swing them up backward to the right until the right hand comes to the height of the shoulders with the palm facing upward and the left hand is in front of the chest with its palm facing inward and the elbow bent, once more holding the imaginary ball. At the same time move your weight to the right foot while looking at the right hand while breathing out.

5 On an inward breath draw the right hand back and place it at the inside of the left wrist then push both hands forward with the left palm inward and the right one outward while bending the left leg, breathing out, and leaning forward with the eyes looking at the left wrist. This is "press" (*ji*).

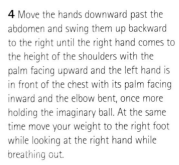

PUSH (AN)

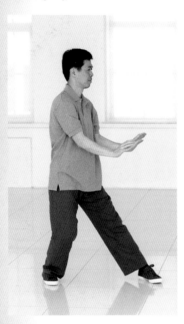

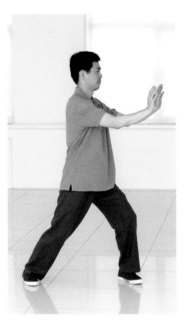

6 Finally breathe in and move the arms forward, a shoulder-width apart, with both palms facing downward, lower the upper body and lean slightly backward while shifting the weight to the right foot and drawing both hands back to the two sides of the waist with palms facing forward and to the ground, breathe out, while eyes look ahead.

7 Push forward and upward with both hands while bending the left leg and leaning forward, still looking ahead. This is "push" (an).

WAVING HANDS LIKE CLOUDS (*YUN SHOU*)

This sequence moves from the far left to the far right and back again in a gentle flowing manner with the hands like floating clouds.

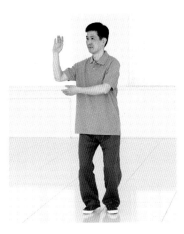

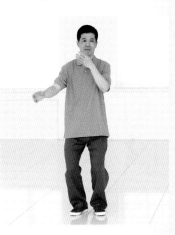

1 Turn the body to the right side with the right hand outstretched and then brought to rest with the upper arm to the right side, held slightly lower than the shoulder, and the elbow bent so the lower arm is upright, palm facing forward. At the same time move the left arm down and then upward toward the right side to lie across the body with the palm turned to face the right elbow. Move the right leg toward the left until standing with the feet close together and knees bent and turn the head to look to the right.

2 Next, with the palm of the left hand facing the body, move the left arm to the left in an upward arc from the shoulder, so the palm passes in front of the face, while the right arm drops to waist level, with the palm facing the body, and rotates upward to the left, while turning the waist to the left and looking in that direction.

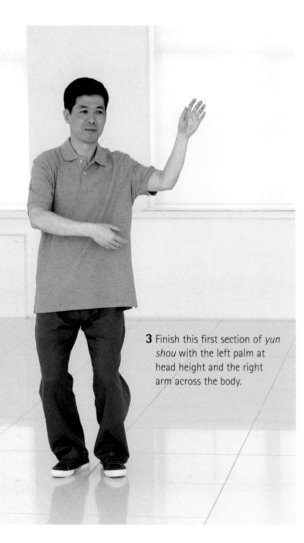

3 Finish this first section of *yun shou* with the left palm at head height and the right arm across the body.

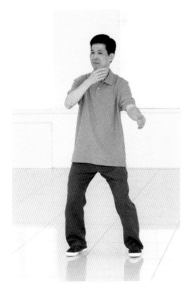
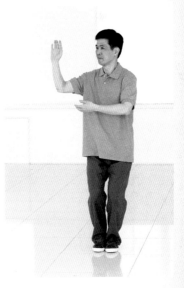

4 From the far left position, move the right arm from the shoulder up and to the right so the palm passes once again in front of the face. At the same time step to the left with the left leg and lower and straighten the left arm, moving it down and to the right, with the waist again turning the upper part of the body until you are once again in the far right position looking to the right.

5 Bring the right arm up so the palm is about face level and drop the left arm to waist height while stepping to the left with the right leg so the feet are together. This completes the second section of *yun shou*. In a full *t'ai-chi* sequence the first part of the movement is then repeated, moving body and arms again from the far left to the far right with the hands moving across like a floating cloud to complete the third and final part of the movement.

SINGLE WHIP (*DAN BIAN*)

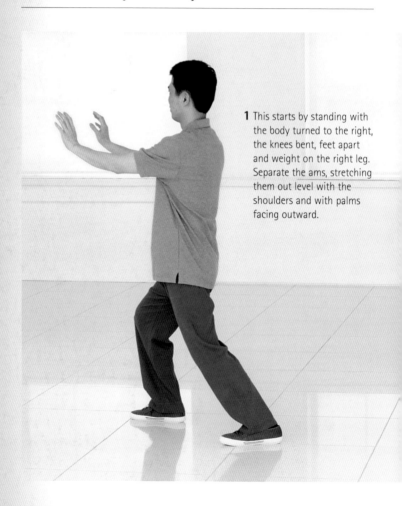

1 This starts by standing with the body turned to the right, the knees bent, feet apart and weight on the right leg. Separate the ams, stretching them out level with the shoulders and with palms facing outward.

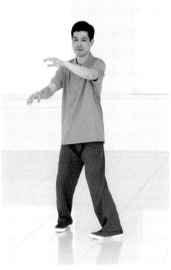

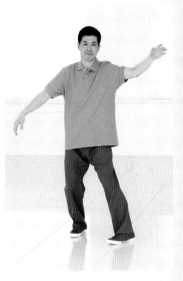

2 Next turn the torso to the left, pivoting on the right foot and drawing the arms across the body at about chest height, lowering the right arm slightly so the hand is at waist height.

3 Once the arms have just reached the left side, draw the right arm back across to the right side and stretch the left arm out, palm facing forward.

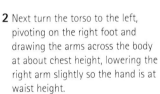

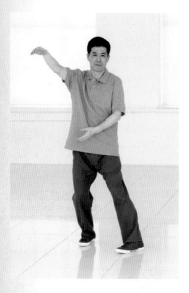 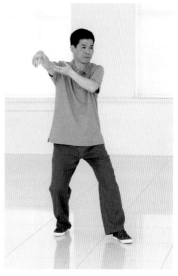

4 As you draw the left arm down and in front of the body, raise the right arm in front of you and to the side.

5 Continue to raise the left arm until it reaches the right arm and at the same time shape the right hand into a beak with the thumb touching the other fingers and all the fingers pointing down. Simultaneously turn the left foot to the left and turn the head to face the same way.

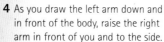

6 Finally, bring the left arm up to face level with the palm facing the face. Step to the side and forward with the left leg while the left hand follows in the same direction pushing forward with the palm facing out. This finishing position is *dan bian*.

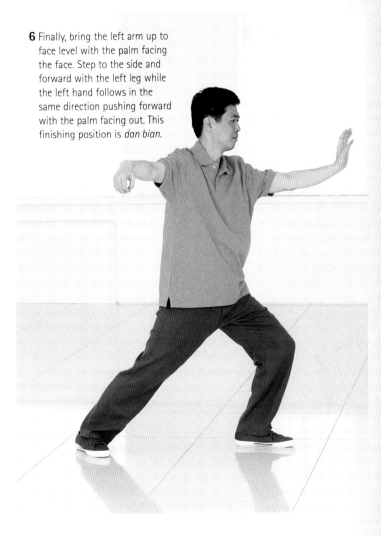

WHITE CRANE SPREADS ITS WINGS
(*BAI E LIANG CHI*)

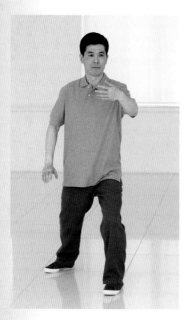

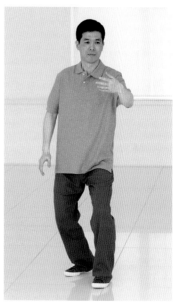

1 From a standing position, turn the right foot to the right and step forward and to the side with the left foot. Raise the left arm out in front of you with the elbow slightly bent and the palm facing the body. Push down with the right palm, with the elbow slightly bent. Face to the left, looking over the left hand.

2 Draw the right foot forward toward the left foot. Twist the right hand so the palm faces the body.

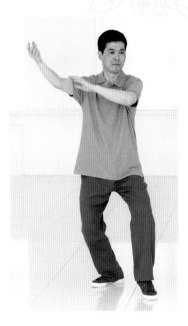

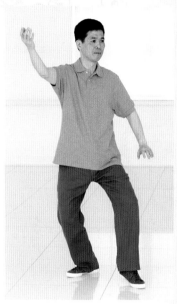

3 With the left leg step slightly to the left with the toes, keeping the heel off the ground. At the same time raise the right arm to shoulder height with the palm facing forward at head height and bring the left arm across so it is level with the right shoulder, palm facing down.

4 Finish by transferring almost all your weight to the back right leg and moving the left arm down to rest along the left leg with the palm down and the chest facing forward. Look slightly to the left. Relax and breathe out as the weight settles down in the back right leg.

THE HEALING POWER OF QI

While exercise therapies like *qigong* and *t'ai-chi* form one of the "eight limbs" of Chinese medicine and can strengthen the *qi*, they also energize the *dan tien* so have a spiritual dimension.

Like the *san jiao* (Triple Burner) the *dan tien* is a nebulous, three-fold entity. While the *san jiao* has a physical function the three levels of the *dan tien* can be equated to the physical, emotional and spiritual aspects of our being. *Dan tien* can be translated as "elixir field" and is believed by some to be the reservoir of *qi, jīng* and *shén*.

THE THREE LEVELS

The lower *dan tien* (at and below the navel)—where the acu-points *qi hai* (CV6) sea of *qi*, and *shen que* (CV8) the spirit gate, can be found—is associated with the Earth and the physical body. Focusing exercise techniques on strengthening this area of the *dan tien* can help control physical illness and strengthen vital energy.

The upper *dan tien*, linked to spiritual aspects of being and heaven, is focused at the crown of the head at the acu-point GV20 *bai hui* (translated as celestial convergence) and at the *yintang* point between the eyes, sometimes called the "third eye."

The middle *dan tien* is linked to the emotional aspects of being and is located at the Heart, which is where the Chinese concept of "heart-mind" resides. The Heart in Chinese medicine is seen as the seat of emotions and thoughts rather than the brain. Focusing energizing exercise routines on the middle *dan tien* is said to heal emotional trauma, mental distraction and worry and to ease stress—an acknowledged cause of illness in Western medical theory.

Using meditation and energizing exercise can thus play a significant part in healing, especially if illness and healing are regarded holistically.

THE THREE LEVELS OF
THE *DAN TIEN*

Upper *dan tien*

Middle *dan tien*

Lower *dan tien*

GLOSSARY

Adrenocorticotropic hormone (ACTH): a hormone synthesized and stored in the anterior pituitary gland, of which large amounts are released in response to any form of stress

AIDS: acquired immune deficiency syndrome

Antiemetic: a substance to combat nausea

Antipyretic: a substance that reduces body temperature in fevers

Arteriosclerosis: a build-up of fatty deposits in the blood vessels leading to narrowing and hardening, and associated with heart disease and strokes

Arthralgia: joint pain

Bì syndrome: literally "pain syndrome," a term usually applied to arthritis-like conditions

Body Fluids: *jin-ye*—one of the five fundamental substances of Chinese theory

Carminative: relieves flatulence, digestive colic, and gastric discomfort

Cathartic: a substance that acts as a more drastic laxative than a purgative

Cervical dysplasia: the enlargement of the cervix by abnormal cells; usually an early stage in the development of cervical cancer

Cervical vertebrae: the vertebrae immediately below the skull

Channels: invisible pathways in which *qi* travels; also called meridians. They appear in and on the body

Cholagogue: stimulates bile flow from the gallbladder and bile ducts into the duodenum

Cholecystitis: inflammation of the gallbladder

Coccyx: a small triangular bone at the base of the spinal column formed from fused vertebrae

Cystitis: inflammation of the bladder

Damp: in Chinese medicine, Damp is considered to be a *yin* pathogenic influence, leading to sluggishness, tired and heavy limbs, and general lethargy

Decoction: a herbal preparation where the plant material is heated in cold water and simmered for 20 minutes to produce an extract

Dan tien: the "elixir field" divided into upper, middle, and lower and associated respectively with *shén*, *jīng* and *qi*

Diaphoretic: a substance that increases sweating

Diuretic: a substance that encourages urine flow

Ensiform: a type of early acupuncture needle shaped like a sword blade

Expectorant: a substance that enhances the secretion of sputum from the respiratory tract so that it is easier to cough up

Febrifuge: a substance that reduces fever

Femur: thigh bone

Fibula: the outer and usually smaller of the two bones in the lower leg between knee and ankle

Fu: the hollow *yang* organs of the body—Small Intestine, Gall Bladder, Large Intestine, Urinary Bladder, and Stomach

Gluteal crease: the horizontal groove which marks the lower limit of the buttock where it meets the top of the thigh

Hepatitis: inflammation of the liver

Huang Di: the Yellow Emperor, who reputedly lived sometime between 4000–2500 BCE. In Chinese legend he was the supreme ruler of the universe, introduced music, medicine and mathematics, writing and weapons. He was the reputed author of the *Yellow Emperor's Classic of Internal Medicine* (*Huang Di Nei Jing Su Wen*), first written down some time between 206 BCE–250 CE. It was the core textbook for Chinese physicians for generations

Hypertensive: a substance that raises blood pressure

Hypoglycemic: a substance that reduce blood sugar levels

Hypotensive: a substance that lowers blood pressure

Inguinal groove: the groove between the pelvis and lower abdomen.

Inter-costal space: the space between each of the ribs

Jin-ye: Body Fluids—one of the five fundamental substances—*jin* refers to the lighter or clear fluids, *ye* to the denser or turbid fluids

Jīng: one of the fundamental substances—the vital essence that is the source of life and individual development

Laxative: a substance that encourages bowel motions

Li Shi Zhen (1518–1583): a renowned Chinese physician and herbalist, author (in 1578) of the *Compendium of Materia Medica* (*Ben Cao Gang Mu*) which details 1,892 vegetable, animal and mineral drugs then in regular therapeutic use. His book on pulse diagnosis (*Bin Hu Mai Xue*) is a classic on the subject

Lochia: the normal discharge from the uterus after childbirth

Lumbar vertebrae: the five vertebrae in the lower back below the thoracic vertebrae

ME: myalgic encephalopathy also known as chronic fatigue syndrome

Medial malleolus: the protuberance at the lower end of the tibia

Oxytocin: a hormone produced by the pituitary gland which increases uterine contractions during labor and also stimulates milk flow

Perineum: the area between the anus and scrotum or vulva

Peripheral vasodilator: a substance that dilates (makes larger) the peripheral blood vessels

Phlegm: in Chinese medicine, disharmony of the Body Fluids produces either external (visible) Phlegm, or internal (invisible) Phlegm

Prostatitis: inflammation of the prostate gland

Pubic bone: the small bones at the base of the pelvis

Purgative: a substance that acts as a drastic laxative.

Qi: the Chinese term for the life force or vital energy of the universe, which is fundamental to all aspects of life. It permeates the whole body and is concentrated in the channels

Radius: the thicker and shorter of the two arms in forearm. The radial pulse is felt where the radius meets the wrist at the thumb

Rubifacient: a remedy which causes redness of the skin by heating the area and increasing blood flow

Sacrum: a triangular bone in the lower back formed from fused vetebrae and located between the two hip bones of the pelvis

Scrotum: the pouch of skin containing the testicles

Shen Nong: the "divine farmer" reputedly lived sometime between 4000–2500 BCE. According to Chinese legend he first taught mankind how to cultivate grains and personally tasted hundreds of herbs to identify their healing properties. He is the reputed author of the *The Divine Farmer's Herb Classic* (*Shen Nong Ben Cao Jin*) which was first written down sometime between 206 BCE–250 CE

Shén: one of the five fundamental substances, equates with "Spirit"

Tāng: "soup"—a Chinese medicinal decoction

Tendonitis: inflammation of a tendon

Tibia: the outer and usually larger of the two bones in the lower leg between knee and ankle

Thoracic vertebrae: the twelve vetebrae making up the central section of the spinal column.

Three treasures: the collective term used to describe *qi*, *jīng*, and *shén*.

Urethritis: inflammation of the urethra (the duct by which urine passes from the bladder to the outside world)

Vulva: the external opening of the vagina

Wei qi: defensive *qi*, which protects the body from invasion by external pathogenic factors. It flows just beneath the skin and is sometimes likened to the body's immune system

Xue: one of the five fundamental substances, equates with blood

Zang organs: the solid *yin* organs of the body—Heart, Liver, Lungs, Kidney, and Spleen

Zang-fu: the term used in traditional Chinese medicine for the complete set of five *zang* (solid) organs and five *fu* (hollow) organs

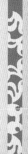

INDEX

ACKNOWLEDGMENTS

AUTHOR'S ACKNOWLEDGMENTS

Penelope Ody would like to thank Sandra Rigby, who originally conceived the idea for this book, and Clare Churly for master-minding its production. The recipes in section five are derived from those originally developed for *The Chinese Herbal Cookbook* (Kyle Cathie, 2000) written by Penelope Ody with Alice Lyon and Dragana Vilinac – whose experience of cooking with Chinese herbs is also gratefully acknowledged.

PICTURE ACKNOWLEDGMENTS

Special photography: © Octopus Publishing Group/Ruth Jenkinson
akg-images/British Library 33. **Alamy**/Aflo Foto Agency/Toshihiko Watanabe 198; /amana images inc./DAJ 135; /Arco Images GmbH 203; /Arco Images/O. Diez 169; /Pat Behnke 128; /Bildagentu r-online 175; /Bildagentur-online.com /th-foto 327; /Bon Appetit/Ottmar Diez 145; /Bon Appetit /Ian Garlick 285; /Bon Appetit/David Loftus Limited 290; /Bon Appetit/Peter Rees 165; /Bon Appetit /Teubner Foodfoto 172; /Catchlight Visual Services /Hermien Lam 361; /Flowerphotos/Carol Sharp 170; /Geoffrey Kidd 149, 181, 183, 200; /IMAGEMORE Co., Ltd. 134, 161; /Mary Evans Picture Library 82; /Neil Palmer 197; /OJO Images Ltd/Sam Edwards 71; /Shoosh/Form Advertising 221; /STOCK4B GmbH 218; /TH Foto-Werbung /PHOTOTAKE 157. **Bridgeman Art Library**/Archives Charmet 19. **Corbis**/amanaimages /Yasuno Sakata 24; /Blend Images/REB Images 44; /Bloomimage 29; /epa/Jack Bow 95; /Randy Faris 6, 125; /Peter Guttman 321; /Image Source 76; /Michael A. Keller 107; /PhotoAlto Michele Constantini 67; /PhotoAlto/Vincent Hazat 98; /Redlink/Chan Yat Nin 90; /Rubberball 105; /Science Photo Library /Adam Gault 111, 118; /Strauss/Curtis 217; /Tetra Images/Jamie Grill 42. **Dorling Kindersley** 137; /Neil Fletcher & Matthew Ward 150; /Steve Gorton 176. **Fotolia**/Arik 57; /Norman Chan 185; /Elenathewise 282; /Thierry Hoarau 136. **Garden World Images**/Gilles Delacroix 138, 168, 204, 209.

Getty Images 13; /Caren Alpert 2; /altrendo images 49; /A. Chederros 102; /China Tourism Press 55; /EIGHTFISH 8, 47, 365; /Neil Fletcher & Matthew Ward 151; /Steve Gorton 143, 164; /Jack Hollingsworth 267; /Jason Hosking 334; /Influx Productions 328; /Jose Luis Pelaez Inc. 112; /Kallista Images 73; /Mike Kemp 343; /Frank Lukasseck 59; /PM Images 81; /Purestock 79; /Howard Rice 211; /Benjamin Rondel 30; /Jochen Schlenker 63; /Stockbyte 68, 114; /Keren Su 50, 60; /Dougal Waters 41; /WP Simon 43; /ZenShui/Eric Audras 37. **Masterfile** 212, 243. **Octopus Publishing Group** 297; /Stephen Conroy 74, 269, 293, 301; /Frazer Cunningham 383; /Will Heap 287, 311; /Mike Hemsley 146, 155, 159, 160, 174, 178, 179, 186, 187; /Janine Hosegood 276; /William Lingwood 275; /David Munns 278; /William Reavell 264, 271, 272, 280, 289, 314; /Russell Sadur 259, 263; /Eleanor Skan 286; /Ian Wallace 244, 250, 253, 304. **Photolibrary**/ Ableimages/Jutta Klee 324; /Botanica 191; /Botanica/Linda Lewis 317; /Botanica/Heather Weston 189; /BSIP Medical/Chassnet Chassnet 117; /Corbis 194; /Creatas 97; /Fresh Food Images/Carl Pendle 307; /Garden Picture Library/Francois De Heel 126; /imagebroker.net/Bao Bao 141, 142, 152, 162; /JTB Photo 65, 206; /Oxford Scientific (OSF)/Geoff Kidd 167; /PhotoAlto/Michele Constantini 122, 193; /Norbert Reismann 249; /Ticket/Ben Pipe 333. **Rex Features**/Garo/Phanie 108. **Wellcome Library, London** 11, 53, 101, 133, 215.

Executive Editor Sandra Rigby
Managing Editor Clare Churly
Senior Editor Lisa John
Deputy Creative Director Karen Sawyer
Designer Cobalt id
Picture Library Manager Jennifer Veall
Picture Researcher Emma O'Neill
Production Manager David Hearn